100 Questions & Answers About Your Child's Obesity

Barton Cobert, MD
Gastroenterologist
BLCMD Associates LLC
Westfield, NJ

Josiane Cobert, MD
Child & Adolescent Psychiatrist
Trinitas Regional Medical Center
Elizabeth, NJ

JONES AND BARTLETT PUBLISHERS
Sudbury, Massachusetts
BOSTON   TORONTO   LONDON   SINGAPORE

World Headquarters

Jones and Bartlett Publishers
40 Tall Pine Drive
Sudbury, MA 01776
978-443-5000
info@jbpub.com
www.jbpub.com

Jones and Bartlett Publishers
Canada
6339 Ormindale Way
Mississauga, Ontario L5V 1J2
Canada

Jones and Bartlett Publishers
International
Barb House, Barb Mews
London W6 7PA
United Kingdom

Jones and Bartlett's books and products are available through most bookstores and online book-sellers. To contact Jones and Bartlett Publishers directly, call 800-832-0034, fax 978-443-8000, or visit our website at www.jbpub.com.

Substantial discounts on bulk quantities of Jones and Bartlett's publications are available to corporations, professional associations, and other qualified organizations. For details and specific discount information, contact the special sales department at Jones and Bartlett via the above contact information or send an email to specialsales@jbpub.com.

The authors, editor, and publisher have made every effort to provide accurate information. However, they are not responsible for errors, omissions, or for any outcomes related to the use of the contents of this book and take no responsibility for the use of the products and procedures described. Treatments and side effects described in this book may not be applicable to all people; likewise, some people may require a dose or experience a side effect that is not described herein. Drugs and medical devices are discussed that may have limited availability controlled by the Food and Drug Administration (FDA) for use only in a research study or clinical trial. Research, clinical practice, and government regulations often change the accepted standard in this field. When consideration is being given to use of any drug in the clinical setting, the healthcare provider or reader is responsible for determining FDA status of the drug, reading the package insert, and reviewing prescribing information for the most up-to-date recommendations on dose, precautions, and contraindications, and determining the appropriate usage for the product. This is especially important in the case of drugs that are new or seldom used.

Production Credits
Senior Acquisitions Editor: Alison Hankey
Editorial Assistant: Sara Cameron
Production Director: Amy Rose
Associate Production Editor: Jessica deMartin
Manufacturing and Inventory Control Supervisor: Amy Bacus
Composition: Glyph International
Printing and Binding: Malloy, Inc.

Cover Credits
Cover Design: Colleen Lamy
Cover Printing: Malloy, Inc.
Cover Images: Top: © Multiart/Shutterstock, Inc.; Bottom left: © Eduardo Cervantes/Shutterstock, Inc.; Bottom right: © Stuart Monk/Shutterstock, Inc.

Library of Congress Cataloging-in-Publication Data
Cobert, Barton L.
    100 questions & answers about your child's obesity / Barton Cobert, Josiane Cobert.—1st ed.
        p. cm.
    Includes index.
    ISBN 978-0-7637-7832-3 (alk. paper)
    1. Obesity in children—Miscellanea. 2. Obesity in children—Popular works. I. Cobert, Josiane. II. Title. III. Title: One hundred questions and answers about your child's obesity.
    RJ399.C6C63 2010
    618.92'398—dc22
                                                                2009038841
6048

Printed in the United States of America
13 12 11 10 09   10 9 8 7 6 5 4 3 2 1

To our parents (who fed us well, perhaps too well).

Contents

You have heard it from the medical profession and have seen it on television, in the street, and at school (and it is true): An epidemic of obesity is striking children and adults in America, and it is taking its toll on our health.

The percentage of obese and overweight preschool children (2 to 5 years old) and adolescents (12 to 19 years old) has doubled, and for children 6 to 11, the percentage has tripled in the last 30 years. About 9 million children over 6 years old are obese, and many more are overweight. This can be physically dangerous for children, as they can develop diabetes, high blood pressure, and other diseases. Being overweight can also produce pressure, teasing, bullying, depression, and other social problems for a child, as "thin = attractive" and "fat = ugly." Society pays with time lost from work and school, mounting health expenses caused by obesity, and other direct and indirect costs.

No one really doubts that this is a problem. Unfortunately, no magic or easy answers are available. We, both as a society and as individuals, need to eat better and less and exercise more. That really is the take-home message of this book. The answer for the child who is overweight or obese lies with the child and his or her family. This book is an attempt to help you and your child handle excess weight.

Your child (and you, if you are too heavy) can get to a normal weight, but this takes self-control, hard work, and a change in lifestyle that is not just for 6 weeks or 6 months; instead, it is forever. The advice in this book is straightforward and simple (but not easy): Eat the appropriate number of calories per day of balanced food and increase exercise.

Your child's health and life are at stake.

We give special thanks to an old and wonderful friend, Steve Shifrinson of the Marlboro, New Jersey school system, who helped with many of the school-related aspects in this book.

PART ONE

Definitions and Measurements

What is the "normal" weight of a person? How is it determined?

If height matters, then how do you account for height in finding a normal or healthy weight?

I heard that waist circumference is important. What does it mean if my child has a large waist size?

More . . .

1. What is the "normal" weight of a person? How is it determined?

The normal (perhaps a better term is "healthy") weight for an individual is actually a function of age, gender, and height. Charts published by the U.S. Centers for Disease Control (CDC) represent the weights and heights for American children. Most of these charts show the healthy weight for a child, although some are actual measurements of weights of children in the United States and represent the "real" weights but not necessarily healthy weights. Several of the charts are included in Appendix B of this book. A complete set of charts from the CDC is available at: http://www.cdc.gov/growthcharts.

Online calculators are also available to do the math for you. This calculator will take your child's gender, age, height, and weight and give you the percentile that he or she is now and what the "ideal" body weight should be: http://pediatrics.about.com/cs/growthcharts2/l/bl_ibw_calc.htm.

The data in the charts are arranged by age and gender and are placed into "percentiles." A percentile is the percentage of the population that weighs a given amount or less. Table 1 shows some examples in graph form.

For example, look at the 10-year-old boy line that is highlighted. If your son weighs 55 pounds, then 5% of all other boys weigh less than he does and 95% weigh more. If he weighs 71 pounds, then half weigh more and half weigh less. If he weighs 102 pounds, then only 5% weigh more and 95% weigh less.

As you can see from this chart, boys and girls weigh roughly the same until the age of 10, or so, when the boys start getting bigger than the girls. These are not

Table 1   Weight percentiles for children.

Percentile	5%	10%	25%	50%	75%	90%	95%
Boy, 5 years	33	35	38	40	44	48	51
Girl, 5 years	32	33	35	39	44	48	51
Boy, 10 years	55	57	63	71	80	93	102
Girl, 10 years	53	57	63	72	83	96	106
Boy, 15 years	94	99	110	124	140	159	173
Girl, 15 years	89	94	102	114	129	151	165

If your 10-year-old son weighs 55 lbs., 5% of other boys his age weigh less and 95% weigh more. If he weighs 71 lbs., half weigh more and half weigh less. If he weighs 102 lbs., only 5% weigh more and 95% weigh less.

normal weights, but the actual weights of American children, as measured by the CDC and published in 2000. Many authorities feel that on the average, Americans are too heavy. Thus, these chart weights may be too high for optimal health.

2. If height matters, then how do you account for height in finding a normal or healthy weight?

Yes, height matters. The charts and calculator previously noted account for height.

An easy way to find the healthy weight for your child has been developed and takes into account both weight and height. It is called the **body mass index (BMI)**. The calculation is a bit complex. It is figured by taking the weight in kilograms (kg) divided by the height in meters squared (m²). This works easily in the metric system but is a little more complicated in the pounds/inches American system.

Body mass index (BMI)

A number calculated from height and weight that is used to determine whether a person is in the "normal" weight, underweight, overweight, or obese range.

The formula is as follows:

$$BMI = \frac{weight \ (pound) \times 703}{height \ squared \ (in^2)}$$

For example, the BMI of a child who is 5-feet and 1-inch (61 inches) tall and weighs 105 pounds would be calculated as:

$$BMI = \frac{105 \times 703}{61 \times 61} = \frac{73,815}{3,721} = 19.8$$

An easier way to find this is by using an already created calculator (see the Resources for some online examples).

The BMI is not in and of itself a measure of **fat** in the body. Other, more complicated ways of doing that, including measuring skin-fold thickness, are available (see Question 8). Nonetheless, the BMI for most people is a very good tool for evaluating excess weight (see Question 6).

3. I heard that waist circumference is important. What does it mean if my child has a large waist size?

Excessive abdominal (stomach, belly) fat has a worse health prognosis than fat distributed elsewhere on the body. A male with a waistline over 40 inches or a non-pregnant female with a waist of more than 35 inches is at a higher risk of developing such medical conditions as **diabetes mellitus**, elevated **cholesterol** and **triglycerides, hypertension**, and **coronary artery (heart) disease**. Thus, it is not just the weight that matters, but also the weight distribution. Weight around the waist is worse than excess pounds in, say, the legs.

Metabolic syndrome is a condition that is sometimes seen in adults. This is cluster of risk factors for heart disease and stroke and includes the following:

Fat

See also lipids. One gram of fat contains and produces nine calories of energy. As an adjective and colloquially, it refers to being overweight or obese.

Diabetes mellitus

A complex disease of small blood vessels and glucose metabolism. It is manifested by elevated levels of sugar (glucose) in the blood. Long-term adverse consequences include kidney failure, cataracts, poor circulation leading to heart attacks, strokes, leg ulcers, and other serious problems.

Cholesterol

A fat (lipid) that is an essential part of the membranes of cells. It is made by the body as well as ingested with food. It is a steroid and is necessary for life, but an excess can produce atherosclerosis leading to vascular and other diseases including heart attacks and strokes.

- Excess abdominal fat
- Abnormal blood **lipids** (fats), including high triglycerides, decreased **high-density lipoprotein (HDL) cholesterol**, and elevated **low-density lipoprotein (LDL) cholesterol**
- **Insulin** resistance/high blood sugar
- High blood pressure
- Elevated markers of inflammation such as blood C-reactive protein

The key problems with the metabolic syndrome are **obesity** and insulin resistance. It is estimated that 50 million people in the United States have this syndrome, which the American Heart Association defines as follows:

- Waistline: men ≥ 40 inches (102 cm) and women ≥ 35 inches (88 cm)
- Elevated triglycerides ≥ 150 mg/dL
- Reduced HDL ("good") cholesterol: men < 40 mg/dL and women < 50 mg/dL
- High blood pressure ≥ 130/85 mm Hg
- Elevated fasting blood **glucose** ≥ 100 mg/dL

Key to treating this is prevention of obesity in children.

After a person has this syndrome, the goals are to lose weight, treat the elevated blood pressure and sugar, increase exercise, and go on a diet low in saturated and **trans fats** and cholesterol.

4. My son's BMI is 19.8. What does this mean?

Here is how to interpret the BMI:

- Underweight = < 18.5
- Normal weight = 18.5–24.9
- **Overweight** = 25–29.9
- Obesity = BMI of 30 or greater

Triglycerides

Lipids or fats composed of three molecules of fatty acid attached to one molecule of glycerol. Elevated levels have been associated with the development of serious medical diseases.

Hypertension

An elevation of the pressures in the heart and arteries, which can lead to severe disease including heart attacks and strokes. Also called high blood pressure.

Coronary artery (heart) disease

A disease of the arteries of the heart in which the deposition of plaque (cholesterol, calcium, and other compounds) progressively blocks the flow of blood to the heart, which can lead to chest pain (angina pectoris) and myocardial infarction (heart attack).

Metabolic syndrome

A medical condition that is a collection of risk factors for serious disease (including diabetes, heart disease, and stroke). The risk factors include high blood (serum) fat/lipid levels, insulin resistance, high blood pressure (hypertension), and elevated markers of infection seen by doing certain blood tests.

Lipids

Fats found in the body and measured in the blood. They include HDL ("good") and LDL ("bad") cholesterol as well as triglycerides. Lipids are one of the three main sources of energy for the body and a building block for many cells. The chemical definition is a solid, greasy carbon-based material.

High-density lipoprotein (HDL) cholesterol

"Good cholesterol." The lipoproteins help carry the cholesterol to the liver for excretion from the body.

Low-density lipoprotein (LDL) cholesterol

"Bad cholesterol." Lipoproteins help to carry the cholesterol from the liver to the rest of the body.

This means that your son has a normal (healthy) weight for his height because his BMI is 19.8. It falls in the 18.5 to 24.9 range.

Appendix B shows BMI charts that are similar to the height and weight charts referred to in Question 2. By using those charts (Page 164), you will find that this BMI for a 15-year-old boy places him in the 50th percentile (one-half of boys have higher BMIs, and one-half have lower BMIs).

It is easier just to calculate the BMI using the formula or calculator. Then you do not have to worry about age and gender.

5. What is the difference between being "obese" and being "overweight?"

In the past, there has been some confusion about terms such as obesity, risk of obesity, overweight, **morbid obesity**, and others. This subject has become much clearer because of a major review of the subject of childhood obesity done by an expert committee under the auspices of the American Medical Association and two parts of the U.S. Health and Human Services Department: the Health Resources Service Administration and the CDC. They reviewed the entire subject of childhood obesity and made recommendations in December 2007 in the journal *Pediatrics*, published by the American Academy of Pediatrics (see Resources). The first objective of the committee was to standardize the definitions used.

Being obese or overweight means having too much body fat compared with the normal or healthy weight. Because a healthy weight is also a function of height, the definitions used now are based on the BMI, which,

Table 2   Healthy range of BMI.

Status	BMI Percentile Range	BMI numbers
Underweight	< 5%	< 18.5
Healthy	5% to 85%	18.5 to 24.9
Overweight	85% to 95%	25 to 29.9
Obese	> 95%	≥ 30
Extreme obesity	> 99%	> 40

as noted previously, is a number calculated from weight and height. Table 2 shows the healthy range of BMI to be in the percentile range of 5% to 85%, corresponding to BMIs between 18.5 and 24.9.

Overweight, using this definition, is a BMI of 25 to 29.9. By using the calculator or tables, you can then take your child's height to see where the cutoff weight is for the healthy category.

You or your child's doctor can use the CDC tables to calculate your child's status. For example, if your son is 8 years old, 49 inches (4 feet 1 inch) tall and weighs 100 pounds, his BMI is 29.3. He is overweight.

Now looking at the table for boys in Appendix B, you will see that the 25th percentile for his age and height is 50 lbs. That is, 1/4 of all boys weigh less than 50 lbs. and 3/4 weigh more. Continuing:

The 50th percentile is 55 lbs.

The 75th percentile is 64 lbs.

Insulin

A hormone that helps to regulate blood sugar by lowering it. Insufficient insulin or lack of sensitivity to insulin can produce the disease diabetes.

Obesity

The condition of being heavier (or having a higher BMI) than overweight and significantly heavier than normal weight. Obesity is defined as a BMI of 30 or higher.

Glucose

A simple sugar (carbohydrate) found in the body and easily measured in the blood.

Trans fats

A specific type of fat—usually solid rather than a liquid or oil—that is made by adding hydrogen to liquid fat. Excess trans fats have been implicated in the development of heart disease and other health problems.

Overweight

A body mass index of 25 to 25.9, which is greater than the normal weight (or body mass index) but less than the obese weight range.

Definitions and Measurements

Morbid obesity

At the upper end of the obese weight range. A body mass index of greater than 35 or 40 (this is not fully standardized). Also, massive or extreme obesity.

The 90th percentile is 72 lbs.

The 95th percentile is 77 lbs.

So, at 100 lbs., he is heavier than 95% of all boys his age and height—this is too much. To get down to the area you want to realistically be at, between roughly 50% and 95%, he would need to drop his weight from 100 lbs. to below 77 lbs. and ideally to around 60 lbs. The available tables can be difficult to use and the ideal weight and BMI for your child may be complex to calculate, but using an online calculator (see the Resources for examples) can give you a quick and easy answer.

6. What is "morbid obesity?"

Several other terms are used in the medical literature to define and classify excess weight. They have not been fully standardized. They revolve around the BMI and are included in Table 3.

Table 3   Terms used to define and classify excess weight.

BMI	Classification	Other Terms
< 18.5	Underweight	
18.5 to 24.9	Normal	
25 to 29.9	Overweight	
30 to 34.9	Obese—Class I	
35 to 39.9	Obese—Class II	
> 40	Obese—Class III	Severe Obesity
40 to 40.9		Morbid Obesity
> 50		Super Obesity

So morbid obesity, super obesity, or severe obesity represent the patient with the heaviest weight and the greatest risk of severe health problems. "Morbid obesity" is an old term and tries to capture the idea that this excess weight is a risk to health and may even be life threatening.

7. Maybe my son is just a bit short and is slow in developing? Do we have to worry now, or can we wait a bit?

It is certainly possible that your son is just in a slow patch of his growth and development and that he will sprout up at some point and drop to a normal weight for his height. You really cannot presume, however, that this will happen. Thus, you should act now if your son is overweight or obese.

A lot of work has been done on fat cells, and how they grow, develop, multiply, and turnover is very important in weight and obesity. Although the work is somewhat controversial and contradictory, the evidence on fat cells supports the notion that obesity as a child produces weight problems in later life. More fat cells are created in children who are obese than in those who are slim. Thus, a child who is fat will have more fat cells throughout life and will have more trouble maintaining a healthy weight. The message is this: Don't let your child become fat because he or she is more likely to remain heavy throughout his or her life.

Data suggest that only 10% of normal-weight kids become obese or overweight adults, whereas about 75% of fat children become or remain fat as adults.

Being heavy can produce some physical problems (see Question 25) that may disappear or lessen if your child's weight becomes normal. Thus, it is not a good idea to wait to see whether your heavy child has a growth spurt and drops to a healthy weight. Instead, get his or her weight down to a good level now.

8. My child is "big boned" (i.e., muscle not fat). Why would he be considered overweight or obese?

That may indeed be the case if your child is very muscular and works out, but some of that muscle may actually be fat. As noted, the BMI does not measure body fat, and your child might benefit from a measurement of body fat. Several techniques are available to measure actual body fat compared with the BMI. These include skin-fold thickness, underwater weight, **bioelectrical impedance**, and others.

Bioelectrical impedance

A highly accurate way to measure a person's body mass. A small electric current, which flows at different rates through fat and fat-free tissues, is sent through the body. When factors such as height, weight, and gender are analyzed with the results, a measure of a person's body fat can be obtained.

Adipose

Fat cells. There are two types: white and brown.

One common, easy, and noninvasive technique is the skin-fold measurement. In this technique, a special instrument is used to measure several sites (e.g., triceps, biceps, abdomen, thigh, and calf) on the body. The skin is pinched into a double layer that includes fat (**adipose**) tissue but not muscle. The thickness is measured at each site. Because special calipers (that must be kept calibrated) and some training in their use are required for consistency, not all pediatricians will perform this test. They may refer you to a fitness or obesity specialist or clinic for measurement.

If, after this measurement, your son has a normal and acceptable level of body fat, there may be no issue with weight. If his BMI and body fat are elevated beyond healthy, however, then we cannot say that he is just "big boned."

LeVon's father:

LeVon is 12 years old and already weighs more than all of his friends. He's very athletic and plays football at school. He's young and still growing and wants to be an offensive guard on the high school football team when he's old enough. He is serious and does well in his classes. I think he'll do fine. He's strong, big boned, and works out a lot. LeVon is not too tall or fast, and that's why he wants to be a guard. He's a great eater, is not picky, and will eat anything we put in front of him. He loves fried food and barbecue, which is very popular here, but he also eats fruits and vegetables. The school nurse told us at the beginning of the year that she was a bit concerned about his weight. We said that he's just big boned, but she said that she was concerned that he is too heavy for his age and height and that not all of his weight is muscle but also fat. That is true, as he does have a "spare tire" around his waist, but for a football guard position, that's good. We're not sure what to do because he is a great kid and is doing fine.

9. How much body fat should my child have, and what is normal?

Broadly speaking, two types of body fat exist: essential fat and storage fat. The body cannot be "fat free." Fat is a normal, necessary component of cells. Cholesterol and triglycerides, for example, are lipids that are required for life but in excess can produce major problems in blood vessels, the heart, and elsewhere. This is essential fat and, in the normal, healthy adult female, makes up about 12% of body weight and in men about 3%. Although unfair, this is the way the body is made.

Storage fat is a way the body stores or stockpiles energy for future use. It is under the skin and inside the body around many organs. Everyone needs a certain amount of storage fat, but an excess is unhealthy. Storage fat in the male is around 12% and in the female is around 15% (yes, still unfair). The ideal percentages of body fat for the population are as follows.

For women:

- Up to 30 years old: 14% to 21%
- 30 to 50 years old: 15% to 23%
- Over 50 years old: 16% to 26%

For men:

- Up to 30 years old: 9% to 15%
- 30 to 50 years old: 11% to 17%
- Over 50 years old: 12% to 29%

The American Council on Exercise has determined that acceptable "fitness" levels of body fat are 21% to 24% for women and 14% to 17% for men. Because this is a bit complicated, it is probably best to stick with the BMI and weight, age, and height when trying to determine what is a healthy weight.

10. What is the difference between white and brown fat cells?

Two kinds of fat (also called adipose) cells exist: white and brown. Their function is to store fat for use by the body as energy but also to keep the body temperature constant and to cushion the organs of the body.

Each white fat cell contains a droplet of fat (lipid). Each cell also contains, on its surface, receptors for **glucagon** and insulin, two **hormones** that play a key role in the regulation of the release of fat into the bloodstream for use by muscle cells for energy.

Glucagon

A hormone that the body uses to regulate blood sugar, helping raise it when it is low.

Hormones

Chemicals produced and secreted by glands, which then act at a distant site in the body.

Brown fat cells are found primarily in newborns and are somewhat different, structurally containing many droplets of fat as well as many **mitochondria**. Their main function is to produce heat. They exist in small amounts in adults, but their role is very limited. Thus, the body needs a certain number of fat cells; however, too many are damaging to one's health.

Recently, findings were published in the *New England Journal of Medicine* on the link between brown fat and healthy body weight. Researchers in Boston, Finland, and the Netherlands studied brown fat in adults, which is found mainly in the neck and around the collarbone (unlike white fat, which is found around the waistline and hips). The researchers found that lean people have much more brown fat than obese and overweight people, that women are more likely to have brown fat than men are, and that brown fat burns many more **calories** and produces far more heat, especially in cooler environments. Perhaps now a medication could be developed to stimulate fat cells to burn fat and produce heat and energy rather than just store the fat. Another approach could be to induce the body to produce more brown fat. Finally, another interesting finding is that it seems to be easier to lose weight by staying in a cool environment rather than a warm one.

Mitochondria

The organs within cells that contain genetic material and produce the cells' energy. Mitochondria have been called the "powerhouse" of the cell.

Calories

Units of energy. Although there is a technical definition (the amount of heat needed to raise one kg of water one degree Celsius at sea level), in the context of this book, it refers to the amount of energy in a food or the amount of energy that a person used.

PART TWO

Demography/ Epidemiology

I have heard people say that there is an "epidemic" of obesity. What does that mean? How bad is the problem in the United States?

11. I've heard people say that there is an "epidemic" of obesity. What does that mean? How bad is the problem in the United States?

The World Health Organization has noted that there are 1 billion overweight adults and 300,000,000 obese adults on a planet of 6 or 7 billion people. There has been about a threefold increase in obesity rates in the developed world (North America, Europe, etc.) compared with 1980. Increases are seen in developing countries as well.

The U.S. Surgeon General has indicated that over 12 million American children (17% of all children in the United States) are overweight.

The U.S. Surgeon General has indicated that over 12 million American children (17% of all children in the United States) are overweight. The prevalence of obesity in 2 to 5 year olds has gone from 5% in the period between 1976 and 1980 to 13.9% in 2004. The prevalence of overweight children has doubled and of overweight adolescents has tripled since 1980. Some 15% of children aged 6 to 19 are obese. The numbers are higher in Mexican-American and African-American adolescents. The data are even more striking if one compares the rates to the 1960s, when only 4% of kids 6 to 17 years old were overweight. Because up to 75% of overweight children become overweight adults, this is not just an isolated problem that goes away as children age.

In a study published in 2009, researchers studied over 8,500 U.S. 4 year olds born between 2001 and 2005. They found that over 18%—about 1 in 5—were already overweight. Differences were noted in various ethnic groups: 31% of American Indian/Native Alaskans, 22% of Hispanics, 21% of Blacks, 16% of Whites, and 13% of Asian 4 year olds were obese. It is shocking that obesity is seen so early—even before these children started school. At a recent Centers for Disease Control (CDC) conference, it was noted that in adults, the prevalence of obesity in the United States increased 37% from 1998 to 2006. The "average" American is now 23 pounds overweight. The cost of treating obesity increased from $74 billion in 1998 to $147 billion in 2008.

The reasons for this appear to relate to the changes in the way we live. Higher incomes seem to have produced a change in the types of food we consume, moving from complex **carbohydrate** foods (fruits, bread, and pasta) to foods high in fat (particularly saturated fat) and sugar. People are also doing less physical work, as machines now do many tasks that humans used to do. In addition, the work week has shortened, and there is more leisure time, as well as an increase in automobiles and public transport, all of which mean that we are expending fewer calories than our ancestors did.

This produces significant disease and disability in the population.

Carbohydrate

One of the three main sources of energy for the body. These are compounds made up of carbon, hydrogen, and oxygen and include sugars, starches, celluloses, and gums. There are several types based on size and shape: monosaccharides, disaccharides, trisaccharides, polysaccharides, and heterosaccharides. They are a key source of energy for the body. Each gram of carbohydrate has four calories.

PART THREE

Causes

My husband and I, along with our parents, are heavy.
Is this a hereditary or genetic problem?

If obesity is genetic, can anything be done
about it?

We have heard that if our daughter is heavy as a baby,
she will never escape being heavy. Is this true?

More . . .

Bardet-Biedl syndrome

A rare familial, recessively transmitted genetic disorder. The clinical characteristics of this syndrome include impaired vision or even blindness, extra fingers, a diminished or missing sense of smell, disease of the heart muscle, abnormalities with the reproductive and urinary systems, mental and developmental abnormalities, and obesity.

Prader-Willi syndrome

A rare genetic disorder affecting one or more genes on chromosome 15. It is characterized by a difficult birth, poorly developed sex organs in the baby, failure to thrive, excess sleeping, speech delay, overeating and obesity, spine curvature, poor muscle tone, learning disabilities, and other abnormalities. The overeating may be extremely excessive, leading to morbid obesity.

Marion's mother:

My 15-year-old daughter is very heavy. She weighs over 220 pounds and is not very tall. We have to go to special stores to buy clothes for her, or I make them myself for her from bed sheets. Our whole family is very heavy. My husband and I are both overweight and always dieting. His brothers and my brothers and sisters are also very heavy. My mom was so heavy that she died during emergency appendix surgery. The doctors said her heart couldn't take the stress of the weight, the infection, and the surgery. I think there's something hereditary about this, and we're going to ask Marion's doctor to see if there is anything to do. I am very concerned.

12. My husband and I, along with our parents, are heavy. Is this a hereditary or genetic problem?

Undoubtedly, an element of genetic inheritance is involved in excess weight. In fact, two syndromes are clearly genetic: **Bardet-Biedl syndrome** and **Prader-Willi syndrome** (discussed below). However, given the enormous increase in obesity in the last 20 to 40 years, it is clear that this is not due to "genetics" alone, since **genes** do not change that quickly. External environmental factors play a role. As some have said, your genes are not always your fate.

The U.S. Office of Health Genomics (a part of the Department of Health and Human Services) has reviewed the effect of genes on excess weight. Evidence for a genetic basis of obesity includes studies of twins, as well as of very obese people who have **mutations** of single genes. The number of people who have an identifiable genetic problem, however, seems to be under 5% of people with excess weight.

Nonetheless, with the mapping of human genes, a Human Genome Obesity Map has been developed and is progressing rapidly. The Office of Health Genomics cites single mutations in 11 genes. These were strongly implicated in 176 cases of obesity. Fifty chromosomal locations relating to obesity have been mapped, and genes that might play a role in obesity have been identified: 426 variants of 127 genes have been associated with obesity. A gene that causes a deficiency of **leptin** (see Question 22) has been found; this deficiency leads to obesity, but is quite rare.

Thus, obesity and genetics are clearly related, and it is likely that, over the years, researchers will identify more genes that are associated with obesity. For many or most cases of obesity, there are complex interactions among multiple genes that affect weight and obesity. It is possible that genomic therapy will ultimately be developed to allow control of the "offending" genes in obesity as well as in many other medical diseases where research is actively underway. It has recently been reported that a gene on **chromosome** 16 called the "fat mass and obesity-associated gene" might be responsible for up to 22% of all cases of common obesity in the general population. It is not yet known what the **protein** that this gene produces (transcribes) actually does, but it has been found that certain variants are associated with increased weight. There is also some link between this gene and diabetes and other components of the metabolic syndrome.

Bardet-Biedl syndrome: This is a rare familial, recessively transmitted **genetic disorder**. The clinical characteristics of this syndrome include impaired vision or even blindness, extra fingers, a diminished or missing sense of smell, disease of the

Causes

Genes

Units of DNA within a chromosome that can produce a protein having a particular function or producing a change in the body.

Mutations

Permanent changes in genes. May or may not produce changes in the individual.

Leptin

A hormone produced by fat cells that seems to play a role in the appetite center of the brain.

Chromosome

Thread-like structures containing genes found in the DNA of a cell. There are 23 pairs of chromosomes in human cells.

Protein

One of the three main sources of energy for the body. Proteins are also prime building blocks for many of the cells in the body as well as for hormones, antibodies, enzymes, and other key compounds. One gram of protein contains four calories.

Genetic disorder

A disease or abnormality in the body due to a problem in the DNA (gene, chromosome) of a person or organism that is inherited.

Hypogonadism

Poorly developed or incomplete sexual organs.

heart muscle, abnormalities with the reproductive and urinary systems, mental and developmental abnormalities, and obesity.

Prader-Willi syndrome: This rare genetic disorder affects one or more genes on chromosome 15. It is characterized by a difficult birth, poorly developed sex organs in the baby (**hypogonadism**), failure to thrive, excess sleeping, speech delay, overeating and obesity, spine curvature, poor muscle tone, learning disabilities, and other abnormalities. The overeating may be extremely excessive, leading to morbid obesity, which is perhaps the most troublesome part of the syndrome.

The "thrifty gene" hypothesis has been developed as a result of this work in genetics. This postulates that in ancient times humans developed genes to store fat so that during times of famine (when hunting or crops failed) the body would have a reserve of energy in the form of fat to get them through these tough times. But now, in the Western world at least, where food is plentiful and we have become much more sedentary, we don't need to store body fat for hard times. Thus, fat storage genes are a remnant of older times that are no longer needed. Yet, although everybody has these genes and cells, not everybody becomes obese. There are clearly other factors in play.

13. If obesity is genetic, can anything be done about it?

No treatment, including gene therapy and genetic manipulation, is available to alter the genetics of a person to correct the disease. Perhaps in the future something will be developed, but now "genetic treatments" do not exist. If your family carries the genes for the

Bardet-Biedl syndrome or the Prader-Willi syndrome, then you certainly should speak with your physician and see a genetic counselor.

14. We have heard that if our daughter is heavy as a baby, she will never escape being heavy. Is this true?

This is true in many children. Currently, a large ongoing study from the United Kingdom, called the Early Bird Study, has shown that between 75% and 90% of the excess weight in children is acquired before they start school—that is, before age 5, or so. If they are heavy at this young age, the data show that they are likely to be heavy at age 9 and even later.

This may be partly due to some earlier suggestions that babies born with low birth weights were at greater risk of becoming diabetic. Parents were thus encouraged to feed their babies with the aim of increasing the child's weight to prevent diabetes. Work now suggests that this is not the case. More recent studies indicate that excess weight produces insulin resistance, which could be a cause or precursor of diabetes mellitus. This is called the "accelerator hypothesis." Many researchers are now suggesting that a major effort be put into making sure that children are not heavy when they enter school.

Currently, a large ongoing study from the United Kingdom, called the Early Bird Study, has shown that between 75% and 90% of the excess weight in children is acquired before they start school—that is, before age 5, or so.

Sandy's mother:

Sandy is 4 years old and she's adorable but a bit pudgy. She's 3-feet 2-inches and weighs 55 pounds. The doctor said that she's overweight but not obese but is afraid that she may become obese. He said she's already over the 95th percentile. She's adorable and is a wonderful kid, though she cries and can throw a tantrum if we don't give her the food she wants. Her brother Tommy, who's 7, is not overweight, and we never had eating issues with him. We've tried to do the same for Sandy as we did for Tommy, but she just won't cooperate. So we've sort of given in and do let her eat candy and cookies more than we should. We do give her fruit and vegetables, but she won't eat them unless we cut up the fruit and add sugar or syrup. The doctor wants us to be more careful about what we feed her, and I guess we'll have to do that but the tantrums are a real problem.

15. But isn't being obese normal? It seems almost everyone is heavy today.

Some data (published in 2005 in the *British Medical Journal*) suggest that parents are less aware of obesity in both themselves and their children. That is, there is a perception now that being heavy is the norm in society and that there is nothing wrong with it. Why is this? There is no clear answer, but the speculation is that because so many people are overweight, we are seeing a combination of denial and desensitization to it.

Not surprisingly in America, there is now something of a pushback to the views expressed by the medical establishment and health agencies against the "epidemic of obesity." This is manifest as the "fat pride" or "fat acceptance" movement. Online blogs and websites are aimed at denying that obesity is as bad as the conventional wisdom has it. Some claim that data show that it is better to be an active obese person (a "fit fatso") than a nonactive normal-weight person (a "sedentary skinny"). Society, it is argued, is adjusting to this normalization with such things as shops aimed at "big" or "large" people as well as government policy now accepting obesity and, in some cases, declaring it to be a disability for which accommodations must be made.

Although people should not be discriminated against, made fun of, avoided, or punished for being heavy, medical evidence overwhelmingly suggests that being too heavy is unhealthy, as noted throughout this book and elsewhere. Although some people may indeed be overweight and live to a ripe old age with few health problems—just as some three-pack-a-day smokers or heavy drinkers can also live to an old age with few problems—this is not the usual case. One can never know in advance who the "lucky" ones will be. The wise course is to keep one's weight down (and not smoke or drink too much).

16. Can any medical diseases cause obesity?

Yes, some diseases—primarily metabolic ones—can cause a child to gain weight. Diseases such as **hypothyroidism** (low thyroid function) and growth hormone deficiency can cause excess weight. Certain drugs (such as certain psychiatric drugs or steroids, whether legal or street drugs) can also cause obesity, but these are unusual in children. Your child's doctor will be able to test for these.

Hypothyroidism

Decreased thyroid function. This can produce weight gain, low energy levels, anemia, constipation, dizziness, hair loss, irregular menses, and other problems.

17. I have heard that viruses can cause obesity. Is that true?

There are data suggesting that adenovirus-36 may play a role in some cases of obesity. One study noted that approximately 30% of obese people had evidence of an adenovirus-36 infection at some point in their life compared with only about 10% of nonoverweight controls. When this virus is purposely given to monkeys, they gain weight. There is evidence suggesting that the virus can cause some **stem cells** to change into cells that hold much more fat than before. The researchers also found a gene in the virus E4 ORF-1 that may be

Stem cells

Cells in the body that are capable of transforming into different, specialized cells upon certain stimuli.

25

Adenoviruses

A group of viruses that affect mainly children. They can produce gastrointestinal and respiratory infections as well as urinary and eye infections.

Anorexia nervosa

A potentially very serious disease that can be fatal. It is characterized by excess weight loss and emaciation even though the patient may perceive him or herself to be "fat." This disease is more common in females than males, and can lead to some patients starving to death.

Orthorexia

A disease in which a person wishes to eat only healthy and pure foods to the point of malnutrition and even starvation. They may avoid the "wrong" or "unhealthy" foods such as those made from animals or fats or those that have preservatives.

responsible for the change. When this gene was blocked, the change did not occur. **Adenoviruses** are a class of viruses that produce various human diseases, including respiratory infections. Some researchers also speculate that a vaccine might be possible against one or more of the viruses to prevent their infections. Others, however, are skeptical of the possibility that obesity is an infectious disease. Research continues.

18. Do eating disorders such as anorexia, bulimia, binge eating, and other diseases play a role in obesity?

Anorexia nervosa is, a very serious disease that can be fatal. It is characterized by excess weight loss and emaciation even though the patient may perceive herself to be "fat." This disease is more common in females than males. These patients may starve to death.

Orthorexia is similar to anorexia, but the reason for the abnormal food-related behavior is not a wish to be thin or a perception of being fat. Rather, these people want to eat only healthy and pure foods to the point of malnutrition and even starvation. They may avoid the "wrong" or "unhealthy" foods such as those made from animals or fats, or those that have preservatives.

Bulimia nervosa is a disease of **binge eating** followed by self-induced purges (vomiting, laxative use, enemas) to get rid of the food just eaten. This can lead to serious heart, kidney, and other diseases as well as depression. Fatal cases have been reported.

Binge eating is characterized by patients eating large quantities of food even when they are not hungry (and even when feeling "stuffed"). Unlike some of the other eating disorders, these patients are often obese and suffer from problems that excess weight causes.

Compulsive eating disorder is a mixed group of symptoms in people who cannot control or stop how much or how often they eat. This has been called an addiction to food. They may eat all day, particularly sugary foods or other foods that they crave. They may be very rapid eaters and go through withdrawal when they stop eating. Patients may feel anxious and panicked while eating and guilty and depressed after eating.

19. How much of obesity is due to the environment and social conditions?

Although there can be a genetic effect in obesity, environment and social conditions play a large role as well. Several things are at work here. Nutrition and diet, as well as calorie intake are felt to be likely factors in excess weight, although this has not clearly been proven. Over the last several decades, the cost of food (as a percentage of a family's income) has dropped to a very large degree. Food is cheaper than in the past and is very plentiful for most of the population. There is a strong trend to eating out and to purchasing prepared foods as more and more women (the traditional preparers of food in the family) have moved into the workplace. Less time and energy are available for preparing food, and the choices in fast-food, food delivery, takeout, and food variety have increased to everyone's delight. Manufacturers and restaurateurs want to please the public and have tended to make foods that are high in salt and fat—though there now is a trend to healthier eating, as people become aware of the role of food and nutrition in the obesity epidemic.

Bulimia nervosa

A disease of binge eating followed by self-induced purges (vomiting, laxative use, enemas) to get rid of the food just eaten. This can lead to serious heart, kidney, and other diseases as well as depression. Fatal cases have been reported.

Binge eating

A disorder in which the patient eats large and excessive amounts of food at periodic or occasional intervals. As these patients usually do not vomit after a binge, they may gain large amounts of weight. Binge eating may be seen in other disorders.

Compulsive eating disorder

A condition in which patients cannot control how much or how often they eat. They often feel anxious or panicked while eating, then guilt or depression after. It has also been called an addiction to food.

Causes

Most people have only a vague idea of the amount of calories and fat in foods. For example, in a fast-food restaurant, a meal consisting of a double burger with bacon and cheese, a large order of French fries, and a medium shake can have about 1,500 calories and over 60 grams of fat. A 5-foot 2-inch tall teenager weighing 120 pounds needs about 2,000 calories a day and should have 40 to 80 grams of fat. This one meal alone accounts for most of the day's intake.

It is rather difficult to calculate exactly how many calories a person takes in per day. A detailed and meticulously kept food diary is the most accurate way to do this.

It is rather difficult to calculate exactly how many calories a person takes in per day. A detailed and meticulously kept food diary is the most accurate way to do this. For the entire population, it is extremely difficult to get an idea of the food or calorie intake because of difficulties in the data collection and large variations among people and groups. There is some data that shows an increase in overall calorie intake in some groups (particularly adolescent females), but there is also some evidence that food and calorie intake has remained more or less the same in some groups of the population. In the United Kingdom, there is even some evidence of a small decrease in overall food intake, as referenced in a 2005 report in *Nutrition Journal*. While obesity rates have been rising, calorie intake has only been shown in some studies to also be rising. Thus, the evidence is somewhat contradictory. In some people, more food eaten is a factor in obesity, but in others, it may not be.

20. What are some other possible causes of weight gain in my child?

Nutrition and Diet (Fat Intake)—Although excess fat intake can lead to obesity, the data, surprising to some, suggest that the average fat intake has not increased and may even have decreased in some groups. For example, males aged 12 to 19 in a survey in the 1970s consumed about 37% of their calories in fat, whereas in 1999–2000, this figure fell to 32%. Some have suggested that overweight children eat larger portions of fat compared with nonoverweight children. Although we clearly have an epidemic of obesity, we don't have a clear increase in fat intake.

The "Built Environment"—There are suggestions that the physical location and environment of a child's school may play a role in childhood obesity. Some feel that a lack of sidewalks, long commuting distances to school, the location in cities or in high-traffic areas, and roads that are dangerous for biking all discourage children from walking or biking to school. These researchers feel that the daily walk or bike ride to and from school promotes good physical health and lower levels of obesity. Another factor may be the availability of unhealthy food. Some research (published in 2008 in the journal *Physiology & Behavior*) found higher levels of obesity in environments with more fast-food restaurants.

Activity—There does not seem to be a large difference between the levels of physical activity of obese/over-weight children and normal weight children. Nonetheless, there is some suggestion that activity levels are now lower than in the past. Some data have suggested that only about one high school student in three attends a daily gym class. Also, data suggest that children and adolescents have increased the time spent watching television, doing computer work, and playing video games at the expense of physical activity.

Racial and Ethnic Influences—Many studies have been done that look at racial and ethnic differences in excess weight. Groups with higher levels of obesity include the following:

- Low socioeconomic families
- Those living in the southern United States
- African American, Hispanic, and Native American adolescents, particularly Hispanic boys and African-American girls

Environmental Chemicals—There have been some research reports that suggest chemicals, so-called **endocrine disrupters** such as tributyltin or bisphenol A (found in food and drink packaging), may alter the body's weight-control mechanisms, particularly if exposure is in a newborn or during gestation. Some have called these chemicals "obesogens." Such chemicals may produce more and/or larger fat cells. Work continues in this area.

Psychological Factors—Some adults and children eat too much in an effort to deal with such psychological factors such as stress, bullying, boredom, or anger. This often runs in families where the children and the parents all react this way.

Food Availability—If your house is stocked with candy, cake, cookies, and other high-fat food, it is not surprising that they will be eaten. Whoever does the shopping for the family should be careful about what is purchased and kept around the house for meals and snacks.

Other Risk Factors—Some work has identified high birth weight, babies taking a bottle to bed, an obese mother, maternal diabetes during pregnancy, and a child's insufficient sleep as risk factors for childhood obesity. It is still not clear what causes excess weight in all childhood cases. More than likely, it is a combination

Endocrine disrupters

Compounds or other external products taken into the body that can interfere with normal body function and may alter a person's weight-control mechanisms. Sometimes casually called "obesogens."

of factors. The presence of several environmental factors perhaps works in a genetically susceptible individual to cause weight problems. Perhaps a small increase
in food intake and a small decrease in physical activity
over months to years slowly add on the pounds.

21. What are the risk factors for obesity in my child?

Certain risk factors have been proposed, based on data
from various studies, for a young child to become
heavy. Some are quite well established (e.g., obese parents) but others less so. The frequently cited risk factors, as published in a 2005 paper in the *British
Medical Journal*, include the following:

- Obese parents
- High birth weight
- Maternal diabetes or excess weight gain during
  pregnancy
- Little physical activity and a sedentary lifestyle
- Insufficient sleep
- Rapid weight gain before the age of 1 year
- Rapid catchup growth from birth to the age of 2 years
- African American, Hispanic, and Native American
  heritage

Other proposed risk factors include the following:

- Lower parental education
- Lower socioeconomic group
- Formula feeding
- Low meal frequency
- Maternal smoking during pregnancy
- Excess television watching
- Bad eating habits (skipping meals, irregular time for
  meals)

- Easy availability of high-fat, high-calorie fast-food
- Parents with sedentary lifestyles and poor eating habits
- Taking a bottle to bed as a baby
- A child with a very emotional temperament, also called an "active personality"
- Food tantrums that result in the parents giving more food to calm the tantrums
- Not walking or biking to school

22. What about metabolism and hormones such as adiponectin, leptin, and ghrelin?

Adiponectin

A hormone produced by fat cells that plays a role in the uptake, production, and storage of glucose, as well as fat metabolism.

Metabolism

The process in which products brought to a living cell are converted into energy and other products that are either used by the cell or excreted.

Endothelium

A thin layer of cells that lines the inside of blood and lymph vessels as well as other body cavities.

Atherosclerosis

A common disease in which plaque (a combination of cholesterol, calcium and other compounds) builds up inside the inner walls of arteries. It can produce obstruction of these arteries leading to heart attacks, strokes and other significant medical problems.

Adiponectin, a protein hormone that is produced by fat cells and secreted into the blood stream, plays a role in the body's uptake, production, and storage of glucose. It also has a role in lipid and fat **metabolism**, weight loss, and protection of the inside (**endothelium**) of blood vessels from inflammation and **atherosclerosis**. It seems to be high in nonobese people and low in heavy people and to act in the brain to increase appetite and to slow energy use during lean times. In some mice studies, high levels of adiponectin produced obesity but seemed to protect the mice from diabetes. Some work has suggested that high levels of adiponectin prevent obesity, improve insulin sensitivity, and work against the development of atherosclerosis. Other work, conversely, has shown that elevated adiponectin levels in older men are associated with higher levels of cardiovascular death. Thus, the role that this hormone plays in obesity, cardiovascular risk, diabetes, and many other diseases is unclear. Pharmaceutical research is underway to develop drugs to alter adiponectin levels, although it is not clear whether we want levels to move up or down.

Leptin is another hormone produced by fat cells. It binds to the **ventromedial nucleus** in the **hypothalamus**, which is the brain's "appetite center," and seems to play a role in providing the **satiety** signal; that is, it tells the brain when a person has eaten enough. (See Question 23.) Obese people may have elevated levels of leptin, suggesting that the body is not responding to this "stop-eating" signal. As an obese person loses weight, the leptin levels drop. The meaning of this is not clear. It may be a signal to the body of a leptin deficiency, which, according to a Columbia University study published in 2005, then acts to bring weight back up. As with adiponectin, many experimental data on leptin exist, much of which are contradictory, and it is not clear whether we want levels to move up or down.

Ghrelin, a hormone produced in the stomach, pancreas, and brain, seems to stimulate appetite. It is high before meals and low after meals. Ghrelin levels are higher in obese people compared with normal-weight people and seem to vary according to the time of day (as many hormones do). Ghrelin may also play a role in determining sleep duration, preventing stress-induced depression, and helping in learning and memory. What role it plays in obesity is unclear, although at least one group has developed an antighrelin vaccine meant to help in weight loss.

A lot of work needs to be done before we can understand the roles of these hormones and figure out how altering their levels with drugs might help in the fight against obesity.

Ventromedial nucleus
The part of the brain found in the hypothalamus associated with satiety. Injury to this area may produce overeating and weight gain.

Hypothalamus
A part of the brain below the thalamus that controls such body functions as sleep, temperature, and appetite.

Satiety
The perception of fullness or satisfaction with food that has been eaten. It is a signal that no more food is needed.

Ghrelin
A hormone produced in the stomach, pancreas, and brain that seems to stimulate appetite.

Causes

PART FOUR

Problems Caused by Excess Weight

How is satiety controlled, and what do I have to do to make my son feel full and to suppress his appetite or cravings?

What is the satiety index?

What is so bad about being fat? What health problems can excess weight cause or worsen?

More . . .

23. How is satiety controlled, and what do I have to do to make my son feel full and to suppress his appetite or cravings?

Satiety is the perception that one is full or satisfied and that no more food needs to be eaten. Satiety is controlled by a complex and not fully understood series of mechanisms centered on the hypothalamus. Several factors seem to produce satiety and include the following:

- A rise in body temperature (which occurs during eating and digestion as energy is required for this)
- The distention of the stomach as food enters
- A sudden increase in blood glucose
- Emotional upset or stress

Certain things stimulate appetite and decrease or override satiety, such as the smell or sight of certain foods.

Various proteins or hormones in the body act on receptors in the brain that signal satiety. Some of these include **cholecystokinin** (a digestive hormone that is also found in the brain), glucagon-like proteins (glucagon plays a role in glucose metabolism), insulin, leptin, ghrelin, and others. This area is not yet well understood.

Some foods seem to be more "filling," such as those high in fiber. Eating these foods during a meal is among various tricks and techniques that are proposed to increase satiety. (See Questions 24 and 90.)

24. What is the satiety index?

Even though the mechanism of satiety is not well understood, attempts have been made to classify foods as those that increase satiety or fullness and those that,

Cholecystokinin

A hormone secreted in the intestines that aids in fat digestion by causing the gall bladder to contract and release bile into the gut as well as causing the pancreas to release digestive hormones. It is also found in the brain as a neurotransmitter where it has entirely different functions.

Some foods seem to be more "filling," such as those high in fiber. Eating these foods during a meal is among various tricks and techniques that are proposed to increase satiety.

on a calorie-for-calorie basis, when eaten stop the desire to continue eating. Some products are even marketed as fullness control foods. To this end, a **satiety index** has been created. It is believed that foods with a high satiety index are more likely to fill you up than those with a low one.

Satiety index
A measure of how much a particular food produces satiety (or fullness).

Little work has been done in this area. These are hard studies to do, as they are quite subjective. No good measure of satiety is available other than asking a person whether he or she is full. It is also not clear whether normal-weight volunteers react the same way as overweight or obese volunteers. Truly, "one man's meat may be another man's poison." Nonetheless, one study by Dr. Susan Holt in Australia had volunteers give ratings to 38 foods every 15 minutes over 2 hours after eating 240 calories of one of these foods. In addition, at the end of the 2 hours, the subjects could then eat whatever they wished. What and how much they ate were also recorded to see whether those who said the test food made them full really ate less food at 2 hours. This was done to validate the subjective satiety score. The authors reported that the satiety scores were consistent with the food eaten at 2 hours and that high-protein, high-fiber, or "wet" foods had higher scores and fatty foods had lower scores.

Here are some of the scores of the satiety index. White bread was arbitrarily assigned a score of 100%.

Lower satiety scores (foods less likely to fill you up): croissant 47%, cake 65%, doughnuts 68%, candy bar 70%, peanuts 84%, yogurt 88%, potato chips 91%, and ice cream 96%.

Higher satiety scores (foods more likely to fill you up): French fries 116%, Special K cereal 116%, bananas 118%, jellybeans 118%, corn flakes 118%, white pasta 119%, cookies 120%, crackers 127%, brown rice 132%, lentils 133%, white rice 138%, cheese 146%, eggs 150%, all-bran cereal 151%, grain bread 154%, popcorn 154%, whole-meal bread 157%, grapes 162%, baked beans 168%, beef 176%, brown pasta 188%, apples 197%, oranges 202%, oatmeal 209%, fish 225%, and potatoes 323%.

Whether this holds true for people who are over-weight, dieting, or eating multiple foods at the same time (as we normally do, of course) is not known.

It may still be worthwhile, however, to use this as a guide in choosing foods when your child diets. The "bad" satiety foods tend to be the unrefined sugar and high-calorie foods, whereas the "good" satiety foods include complex carbohydrates, fruits, and grains. The study is in the *European Journal of Clinical Nutrition*.

25. What is so bad about being fat? What health problems can excess weight cause or worsen?

This year, more than 300,000 Americans will die from illnesses related to excess weight and obesity. Obesity contributes to heart disease, the number-one cause of death in the United States. Excess weight also leads to an increase in the number of people suffering from type 2 diabetes. At least 17 million Americans have diabetes, and another 16 million have **prediabetes**. Each year, diabetes costs America $132 billion. It can lead to eye diseases, cardiovascular problems, kidney failure, and early death.

Prediabetes

An abnormality of glucose metabolism and handling that may be a precursor to or early sign of diabetes.

Some of the diseases and problems associated with obesity in children and adults include:

- Negative stereotyping
- Discrimination
- Teasing and bullying
- Social marginalization
- Low self-esteem
- Depression
- Negative body image
- Stigma
- Prediabetes and diabetes (type 2)
- Heart disease and high blood pressure (hypertension)
- Lung and breathing problems, including **asthma**
- **Hyperlipidemia** (excess fat in the blood, which can obstruct the arteries)
- **Sleep apnea** (pauses of 10 seconds or more in breathing while asleep) and other breathing problems
- Bone conditions (e.g., **flat feet**; **slipped cap femoral epiphysis**, a serious problem where the top of the femur slips out of its place in the hip bone; and **Blount's disease**, abnormal bowing of the legs)
- Gastrointestinal diseases
- Early puberty
- Hygiene problems
- **Hepatic steatosis** (fatty liver)
- **Cholelithiasis** (gallstones) (some studies have shown that up to one-third of all cases of gallstones in children are accounted for by obesity and that the risk for gallstones is four times greater in 14- to 20-year-old obese girls compared with normal-weight girls)
- Menstrual abnormalities
- Balance problems
- Some studies have suggested that obese children may grow up to have lower incomes, higher poverty rates, lower marriage rates, and fewer years of education

Asthma

A common disease of the breathing tubes (airways) in which reversible narrowing occurs producing difficulty in breathing. It can range from mild to severe and can be fatal.

Hyperlipidemia

An excess of one or more lipids in the blood that can lead to heart disease, strokes, and other medical problems.

Sleep apnea

A disease seen during sleep in which the patient stops breathing for 10 seconds or more causing the patient to wake up.

Flat feet

A medical condition in which the arch of the foot collapses, causing the entire sole of the foot to be in contact with the ground. There is some data that people who are overweight or obese are at greater risk of developing flat feet.

Slipped cap femoral epiphysis

A rare but serious problem that occurs in children where the top of the femur slips out of its place in the hip bone. It is seen most commonly in obese adolescent children.

Blount's disease

An abnormal bowing of the legs that occurs in children. While the exact cause is unknown, obesity is one risk factor for this condition.

Hepatic steatosis

A condition where excess fat builds up in liver cells. It can be caused by obesity, diabetes, or excessive use of alcohol. Also called fatty liver.

Cholelithiasis

A disease in which there are stones in the gall bladder and/or common bile duct.

Some of these will become problems, usually only after many years of obesity (e.g., gallstones, heart disease, diabetes), and do not represent problems today in an obese child. Even as kids, however, obese children may have elevated blood cholesterol, high blood pressure (hypertension), and abnormal glucose tolerance/metabolism (prediabetes). These are risk factors for heart disease later in life. One study of 5 to 17 year olds, cited on the Centers for Disease Control (CDC) childhood obesity website, found that 70% of obese children had at least one risk factor, and 39% of obese children had two or more.

Others problems, however, are acute and can affect the child now: early puberty, bone conditions, and the stigma issues (bullying, body image, social marginalization, etc.). This list represents yet another set of reasons to help your child get to a normal weight.

26. Can obesity produce psychological problems?

Yes, obesity and being overweight have been associated with low self-esteem in children and adolescents. This can produce a vicious spiral of further eating, further lowering of self-esteem, and other problems such as depression and hopelessness. Such a child may do poorly at school, cry too much, not sleep well, and be emotionally flat. She may have few friends and be socially isolated. She may be bullied, teased, or threatened by others in school or on the street. This can lead to learning problems and poor school performance. Sometimes your child may try to mask these issues or hide them from you. If you think there is an issue at school, speak to the teacher and other staff members if needed (school nurse, administrator, principal). Understanding the problem is critical.

Jack's mother:

Jack is 8 and we are tearing our hair out. We don't know what to do. He is 4-feet 2-inches and weighs 140 pounds. The doctor said he is massively obese, and I guess she is right. Jack knows he has a problem and tries not to eat too much but doesn't seem to be able to stop himself. He eats only fast-food and junk food. We try to give him vegetables and fruit and good things, but he won't eat them. I think he sneaks food into his room, and we know he eats candy and bad things at lunch. We give him good lunches to take to school, but he trades them away for other things that aren't so good. The vending machines in the school sell candy and cookies and sugar drinks. We know this is bad for him, and the doctor wants us to see a nutrition specialist at the medical school since she said the blood test she did showed his cholesterol was too high and that she's afraid he may become a diabetic. Maybe he'll outgrow it, but we're going to go see the specialist. We don't know what they can do though. Jack does what he wants.

27. I do not want my son weighed at school or in public because he is ashamed of his weight and is called "fatty" and worse. How can we handle this?

The role of schools in the issue of childhood obesity is changing, though slowly. For many years, the schools did not deal with issues of obesity and even did things that worsened the problem. In fact, many schools had and still have contracts with manufacturers to sell and promote soft drinks, fast-food, and candy. In an Institute of Medicine report in 2005, 38% of elementary schools, 50% of middle schools, and 72% of high schools surveyed had contracts for soft drink sales in the school, with 91% of the schools receiving a cut of the sales. Many schools also permitted advertising and

Obesity and being overweight have been associated with low self-esteem in children and adolescents. This can produce a vicious spiral of further eating, further lowering of self-esteem, and other problems such as depression and hopelessness.

promotions to increase sales. In addition, many schools have been cutting back on physical education. In 2000, a survey showed that only 8% of elementary schools, 6% of middle schools, and 6% of high schools had physical education each day for the students.

Some schools are now checking the height and weight of students each year in an effort to track and help control weight problems. Usually this is done in a setting that minimizes embarrassment. If you or your child are concerned about this being done in front of the other children, however, make an appointment with the school administration or nurse, preferably early in the school year, to see whether measurements are taken in public (for example, bringing each grade to the gym all at once to check all of the students).

Your child's sensitivity to being weighed in school is a call for action. If this is the first sign of an issue, discuss it with your child in a nonthreatening, sympathetic way to explore how to start a program to lose weight.

PART FIVE

In the Doctor's Office

When should we seek medical advice for our child's weight problem?

Our daughter's weight is a problem. We are seeing the doctor next week. What will the doctor ask?

What will the physical examination and medical assessment look for?

More . . .

28. When should we seek medical advice for our child's weight problem?

You have already made the first step by realizing that there is a problem. Presumably, your child is also aware. If your child is obese (Body Mass Index [BMI] > 30) or is in the high-overweight range, you should seek medical advice. If her weight is on the way up—more than is appropriate for her age and height—even if she is not quite in the obese category yet, advice is worth seeking. If your child has tried to lose weight on her own and not succeeded or if she is concerned in any way, seek medical help.

29. Our daughter's weight is a problem. We are seeing the doctor next week. What will the doctor ask?

Your daughter's pediatrician has likely been following her height and weight and has spoken to her and you about it during your regular visits. If not, you should certainly ask the doctor about your daughter's excess weight. You might also want to ask him to refer you to a specialist in childhood weight problems. The doctor will do a complete overview of your child's health. The questions will depend on your child's age and will include the following:

- A history of the prenatal period, birth, postnatal period, and childhood nourishment (including breast-feeding)
- Parents' medical history with attention to diseases that might be due to excess weight as well as a weight/height history of the family (parents, siblings, and relatives)
- A developmental history of your daughter with heights, weights, and milestones since birth (if available)

- Your daughter's medical history, illnesses, hospitalizations, and (if past puberty) menstrual abnormalities
- Medications (if any)
- Sleep problems such as snoring, restless sleep, and mouth breathing at night and during the day. Problems such as fatigue in spite of a "good night's sleep," hyperactivity, and inattention at school. This may be suggestive of sleep apnea (see Question 32).
- Eating habits at home and school, eating out, snacking, and so forth
- Your daughter's social history, including family history (and eating habits and customs), smoking, drug use (licit and illicit, including marijuana and alcohol), and so forth
- School history, including eating habits and physical education participation
- Activity, including exercise, physical activity, and how she gets to school
- Identification of possible risk factors for obesity, as well as smoking, alcohol use, early sexual experimentation, poor diet, and lack of exercise
- Medical review of body systems to look for symptoms that might be due to excess weight (e.g., shortness of breath, heartburn, and joint pains)
- Psychiatric history (stress, anxiety, depression, etc.)

30. What will the physical examination and medical assessment look for?

The physical exam will look at the effects on the body of the excess weight. Usually a complete physical exam will be done on the first visit. In addition, particular attention is paid to problems associated with excess weight:

- Examination of the neck to see whether the thyroid is enlarged (looking for hypothyroidism—low thyroid function)

- Skin exam for dry skin, yeast infections, or irritations in moist skin-fold areas, such as in the groin
- Chest/lung exam looking for wheezing, asthma, or other breathing problems
- Heart exam looking for abnormal rhythms, fast heart rate, high blood pressure, and other possible problems
- Abdomen exam looking for enlargement of the liver (fatty liver)
- Joint abnormalities and pain (knee, hip, ankle, and feet)

31. What behavior assessments will the doctor do on my child?

The doctor will look for any possible psychiatric problems that may be a result of the excess weight, such as anxiety, depression, low self-esteem, and stress as well as any possible underlying primary psychiatric or mental disorders. In addition, the doctor will look for psychiatric issues that might be a cause of the weight problem, such as atypical depression or **post-traumatic stress disorder** (e.g., after sexual abuse a girl may increase her weight unconsciously to become less attractive).

The assessment will also look for alcohol and substance abuse problems and will evaluate whether the child or adolescent is developing appropriately and whether he is involved in age-appropriate activities within his social network. Certain psychological tests can be administered if the physician feels that this is appropriate.

32. What is sleep apnea? Why is this a problem?

Sleep apnea, a disorder in which the patient stops breathing for an interval of at least 10 seconds during sleep, can be seen in obese children and adults. This is

Post-traumatic stress disorder

A psychiatric condition that follows a major traumatic event. A variety of symptoms can be produced including anxiety, fear, flashbacks of the event (which are often very intense), difficulty sleeping, irritability, anger, and excessive reactions to being surprised or startled.

The assessment will also look for alcohol and substance abuse problems and will evaluate whether the child or adolescent is developing appropriately and whether he is involved in age-appropriate activities within his social network.

not a minor problem and can, in some patients, produce very serious health consequences, particularly in those patients who are significantly obese. Sleep apnea produces lower oxygen levels and usually causes the person to wake up. This can happen many times during the night, producing a very unsatisfactory night's sleep. During the night, the child may snore, have difficult or labored breathing, get up frequently, and breathe through the mouth (producing complaints of dry mouth on awakening). Your child may also have other sleeping difficulties such as perspiring excessively, wetting her bed, having nightmares, and sleeping in strange positions.

In the morning, this can leave the person tired and unrefreshed and make getting up difficult. Thus, this can be a problem during both the night and the day. Sleep apnea is seen more commonly in middle-aged people but can be seen in obese adolescents. Some studies suggest that over 90% of obese children have sleep disorders, and one study estimated that 7% of obese children may have sleep apnea.

Some children may fall asleep during school, producing significant learning and social problems. Sleep experts feel that the normal and appropriate range of sleep times should be as shown in Table 4.

The daytime symptoms may be incorrectly attributed to some other problem such as hyperactivity problems (**attention deficit/hyperactivity disorder**) unless a careful history is taken. The diagnosis is made in a sleep laboratory by doing a sleep test (polysomnography). Your child will stay overnight in the laboratory, and muscle, brain wave, breathing pattern and rate, and other tests are followed throughout the night. The

Attention deficit/ hyperactivity disorder

A behavioral disease usually seen in children characterized by impulsiveness, over-activity (hyperactivity) and poor attention/ concentration.

Table 4 Normal range of sleep times.

1.5 to 3 years old	12 to 14 hours a night
3 to 5 years old	11 to 13 hours a night
5 to 12 years old	10 to 11 hours a night
Teenagers	9 to 9.5 hours a night

test is painless and noninvasive. Some medical centers have developed systems in which these tests can be done at home rather than in the sleep laboratory.

The primary treatment for sleep apnea is weight loss. Severe cases can be treated with surgery to remove the tonsils or adenoids if these are considered to be the cause. Another treatment involves the use of a machine (called a C-PAP machine) to keep the breathing tubes open during sleep. A sleep specialist may need to see your child.

33. Should any laboratory tests or x-rays be done when my daughter sees her physician?

Routine laboratory tests, including urinalysis, screening blood tests (blood count, liver tests, and urine function), and tests for thyroid problems, may be done. If any problems are evident or suspected, additional tests can be performed, such as a chest x-ray or breathing tests (pulmonary function tests) for asthma or other lung problems, a glucose tolerance test (testing the blood sugar level over 3 to 5 hours after drinking a test drink with a known amount of sugar), and scans for thyroid function.

Your child's physician will determine which, if any, of these tests are required.

34. Is this a family problem or just my daughter's problem?

It is a family problem in one or several senses. Obviously, being heavy is your child's problem. She has to live with it every day and suffers from its consequences, both now and in the future if she remains obese. The family will suffer if she suffers, since her troubled behavior cannot be healthy. This is a family issue if other siblings or the parents are also overweight or obese and is a call for action, as the negative effects on health and well-being worsen over time.

It is likely that resolution of your child's weight issues will not be done on her own but will require active help and support from the entire family. Changes in certain eating habits and customs might be necessary. This is not a minor issue and will cause major health and social problems in the future if they are not present already.

35. I was fat as a child but am not any more. Is this just a stage that my daughter will outgrow?

Maybe, maybe not. Since the data suggest that as many as 75% of fat children become fat adults, the odds are not good that your child will resolve this problem on her own. Active intervention is required. In your specific case, if your child's metabolism is such that she is obese for only a short period during development, then maybe she will indeed outgrow her weight problem and become a normal-weight adult. On the other hand, if this is not the case, you won't know until it is too late. At this stage, waiting would not be a good idea. If she does not grow out of it, she will find it harder to lose weight later in life. You should begin work with her now to control her weight.

36. What is the likely course if my child does not "grow out of it"?

A study done in 1989 by the Department of Pediatrics at University Hospital in Linköping, Sweden, was a 40-year follow-up of adults who were heavy as children. They entered into the study as children between 1921 and 1947. Nearly half (47.5%) remained obese as adults. Children overweight at puberty had higher than expected morbidity (illness) and mortality over the course of their lives. A Harvard study with a 50-year follow-up showed that obese boys aged 13 to 18 had twice the death rate from cardiovascular disease in adulthood than nonobese boys.

Being heavy as a child means that there is a strong chance of being heavy as an adult; being heavy as an adult has very bad health consequences, causing disease and even death.

37. In our culture and ethnic group, nothing is wrong with being heavy. This has always been that way. Why is there a problem?

As noted in Question 25, severe negative consequences of being obese can occur even if this is common in a culture or ethnic group and even if being obese is felt to be a good thing. The health data are hard to argue with, and the health problems that develop can be severe, debilitating, and even fatal.

Given the changing views of obesity and the current popular cultural and social bias in favor of being thin, cultures and ethnic groups that once looked on "bigness" as being good may not still take this same view.

Cindy's stepmother:

Cindy is 17 and has a major weight problem. She's 5-feet 2-inches and weighs 230 pounds. She can hardly walk and is short of breath when she goes more than a block. The doctor said she has early diabetes. She doesn't have her periods regularly, which the doctor said is due to her weight. She also gets skin rashes under her breasts and on her thighs between her legs. She's been badly teased and bullied in school and doesn't want to go. We have to force her to go to school. She's depressed and not doing well in class at all. She's been on every diet there is but hasn't really lost weight. She'd stay on the diet for a couple of weeks but then would start eating again and gain it all back and more. We tried the meals you order in, but she would cheat and eat more than what they send. We're going to send her to a camp for overweight kids this summer. At least she'll be active. She doesn't want to go, but we're forcing her. We also have an appointment with a surgeon after the summer to see if he can put in that stomach band we heard about and that Cindy's doctor said we should consider. I don't like the idea of surgery, but I'm not sure I see too many other things we can do.

PART SIX

Prevention

My son is at a healthy weight now but still needs to have preventive behavior against obesity. Why?

38. My son is at a healthy weight now but still needs to have preventive behavior against obesity. Why?

As noted in the previous questions, many pressures are pushing children to gain weight, including the following:

Vigilance in the future is the main thrust of the prevention plan. If your son is overweight, he should develop and implement a plan to drop the pounds to reach the normal, healthy weight category.

- Society suggesting that being overweight or obese is not a bad thing
- Less physical activity in the schools and in daily life
- Availability of high-fat, high-calorie fast-food and other less-than-ideal eating habits
- Heredity (if you or your spouse or families are heavy)

For these reasons, it is a very good idea to develop and maintain an obesity-prevention program for your son, particularly if he has some of the risk factors noted in Question 21. If he is not overweight now, then his habits are probably healthy, and no major changes are necessary. Vigilance in the future is the main thrust of the prevention plan. If your son is overweight, he should develop and implement a plan to drop the pounds to reach the normal, healthy weight category.

PART SEVEN

Treatment

What is an overview of the treatments
available to help our daughter achieve and maintain
a healthy weight?

If our daughter is in the normal range,
what should we do to keep her from getting heavy?

What is involved in the dietary assessment
and how is it done? What do I need to know about
my daughter's eating?

More . . .

39. What is an overview of the treatments available to help our daughter achieve and maintain a healthy weight?

Several aspects to the treatment of weight problems are summarized briefly here and then discussed in more detail in later questions and answers. First, define where your daughter is on the BMI scale: normal, overweight, or obese. Treatment varies depending on the group in which she falls.

Any treatment should involve your family and environment as well as your daughter. It should also involve your daughter's pediatrician and/or other healthcare professionals. The goals have to be reasonable and positive. You and your child cannot set unachievable weight-loss targets, as this will be very discouraging and may prevent any weight loss at all. Excess weight loss may also harm normal development. Each child is different, and an individualized program should be developed for your daughter. For example, in some cases, it may not be necessary to go on a weight-loss diet if the child is still in growth mode and normal development will help in attaining a normal and healthy weight.

- Diet—Clearly, a good diet and eating pattern are necessary. You and your child may want to develop this on your own by reading books and Internet sites, or you may want to work with her pediatrician and possibly with a dietitian or nutritionist.
- Exercise and physical activity—This may be simple such as walking to school or may be an active exercise program.
- Behavioral changes—Attitudes will need to change, and clear attention will need to be paid to what is eaten and when.

- Medications—No drugs are approved in the United States for childhood obesity, although some exist for adult obesity. These are usually reserved for the more severe cases.
- Surgery—Clearly, this is a last resort that is used only in the most extreme and severe cases.

For healthcare practitioners, an expert committee of the American Academy of Pediatrics in 2007 developed and published the concept of staged diagnosis, assessment, and treatment (see Resources).

This scheme sets up three categories for children based on BMI percentiles: the normal group (5% to 84%), the overweight group (85% to 94%), and the heavy group (>95%). In Question 40, we first discuss the normal group, for which prevention is the goal.

No matter which group your daughter falls into, weight control is a chronic effort. It is not a one-shot deal whereby she loses weight (if she's too heavy), declares victory, and goes back to the eating habits and behaviors that made her heavy in the first place. It requires a lifelong lifestyle that will keep the weight at a normal level.

40. If our daughter is in the normal range, what should we do to keep her from getting heavy?

Your daughter falls into the first group, the 5th to 84th percentile range for BMI. Prevention is the goal here and is probably the easiest to do. It is more difficult to lose weight than to maintain it, although both will involve behavior changes. Keep in mind that the "normal" percentile range is very wide. If your daughter is, say, at 80%, then she would not need to gain much weight to reach 85% (overweight), whereas a child at 30% or even 60% has much more leeway, needing to gain a lot more weight to hit 85%.

In this group of children, you (the parents), your child, and her pediatrician should conduct an assessment of these key risk factors:

- Is there a family history of obesity, diabetes, thyroid disease, heart disease, and other health concerns?
- What is your daughter eating? Is she following the dietary recommendations from the U.S. Department of Agriculture's food pyramid (www.mypyramid.gov)? These are discussed later.
- Is there too much fast-food and eating out? Is her diet balanced?
- How many sugary drinks is she consuming a day?
- Does she get appropriate exercise? Does she walk to school and have regular gym classes at school or extracurricular gymnastics, dance, or some other physical activity?
- How much television does she watch, and how many hours is she seated in front of the computer?

This inventory assessment about your daughter should be easy to administer. It will allow you to see where improvements can be made so that weight never becomes an issue. The following questions and answers cover the specifics of the program for dietary assessment and developing a new eating plan, behavior, and exercise.

41. What is involved in the dietary assessment and how is it done? What do I need to know about my daughter's eating?

There are several ways of doing a dietary assessment. Some are formal, and some are informal. They may be done either retrospectively (looking at what your child has eaten) or prospectively (recording what your child eats over the next several days or week).

The informal methods involve questioning or writing down what your daughter remembers (or what you remember her) eating. In general, this method does not work well, as people do not include everything they ate (whether deliberately or just forgetting). This method is very inaccurate for food that has been eaten more than 24 hours ago. So if this method is used, it should be done at the end of each day, every day. Another similar recall method uses a checklist in which your daughter marks off what and how much she ate. This can be useful as it prompts one to remember.

More accurate assessments can be had in a prospective (moving forward) way in which your daughter records everything that she eats at the time that she is actually eating. It can be done by estimating portion size or amounts eaten and drunk or by actually weighing the food eaten or looking on the package to record the precise calories listed on the label. In very formal or experimental settings, photographs or videos are made of everything consumed.

When your daughter visits the doctor or dietitian, a very careful, detailed history will be taken of a typical week's diet. The doctor might ask her to keep a diary of everything she eats (snacks and drinks, of course, are included). The dietitian or physician will then analyze and quantitate the diary, and an analysis of the balance (fat, carbohydrate, and protein) will be calculated, along with the calories consumed per day.

The recording should cover these things:

- What is eaten and drunk at home and outside (including the school cafeteria and fast-food) both alone or with friends and family as well as takeout foods.
- Drinks consumed, particularly sugary drinks, including juices and energy drinks. Amounts (cans, cups, ounces) are needed in detail.
- What was eaten for breakfast, lunch, and dinner plus snacks and "grazing" (always nibbling on something).
- Portion size. This should be measured or detailed where possible, and if not, it should be estimated.

Some teenagers have used other ways, including instant messages, Tweeting, texting, e-mail, and voice recordings, to record what they eat. Use whatever works best.

42. Are these methods accurate? My daughter says that she eats like a bird but is very obese.

Well, there are parakeets and there are eagles—they eat differently! Obviously, the accuracy depends on recording completely everything consumed, including those two French fries swiped from a friend's burger platter or the candy bar purchased from the vending machine on the way home from school. Portion size matters also, and that can be particularly hard when the food is taken from, say, an open bowl of potato chips rather than a 1-ounce bag where the quantity is clearly known.

People tend to undercount rather than overcount— whether deliberately, accidentally, or unconsciously.

People tend to undercount rather than overcount— whether deliberately, accidentally, or unconsciously. This is usually not frank dishonesty but rather is simply because few people are obsessive about recording and noting what they eat and drink.

Of course, you and your daughter must be scrupulously honest in the counting and recording if you are to get an accurate calorie count. Cheating doesn't help here because you can't fool the body!

43. Our daughter really is obese and needs to lose weight. How much should she lose?

If your daughter is in the overweight or obese category, then a goal should be set to get her to her healthy weight. Because the range of "healthy" weights (5th to 84th percentile) is rather large, (see Question 39), a wide range of weights can be aimed for. Many of the experts do not talk as much about weight now as about BMI. The goal is to move from obese to overweight to normal and then to the middle or lower parts of the normal range. When your daughter steps on the scale, however, she does not see her BMI; she sees her weight in pounds.

The goal should be reasonable and realistic and expressed in pounds. If your daughter is, say, 16 years old, 5 feet tall, and weighs 160 pounds (BMI of 31.2, which is in the obese range and above the 95th percentile) and if she wants to move to the 85th percentile, a weight loss of about 32 pounds to a weight of 128 pounds is necessary. This large weight drop will not happen quickly or easily. Diets that produce weight loss rapidly are unhealthy and usually involve a loss of body water—not body fat—and the weight will return when she goes off the diet. A realistic weight control program aims for a 1- to 2-pound weight loss each week. This would take about 4 to 8 months for the 32-pound weight drop. But even that may sound depressing and unattainable to her.

A good strategy that will make the weight loss seem less daunting is to set an intermediate goal or two.

For example, if the weight she needs to lose to reach the 84th percentile (BMI of 25) is very large, rather than moving there directly as the goal, move to an intermediate BMI of, for example, 28 or 29. This is a weight loss of 15 pounds to about 145 pounds—still overweight but not obese. This is feasible in 2 to 4 months. At that point, another intermediate goal of 15 more pounds—to about 130 pounds—is a BMI of just over 25. Thus, she would be on the upper border of the healthy weight range (<25) in another 2 to 4 months.

You can also aim for a slower weight loss of 5% to 10% of her starting weight over 6 months. She would aim for a loss of 8 to 16 pounds over 6 months, which is about one-fourth to one-half pound a week. This is a bit more modest than the example set above of 15 pounds in 2 to 4 months. Which route she chooses is a question of her willingness to make larger or smaller changes in her diet, to exercise, and to change her attitude and lifestyle. Discuss her choices with her physician and/or nutritionist or dietitian.

By making moderate goals and avoiding very low-calorie diets, the likelihood of success will be greater. The bottom line is this: pick a weight goal that is reasonable for step 1. This will bring her down in a steady way over a reasonable period of time. She can use the weight charts in Appendix B or the calculator mentioned in Question 1 to look for her preferred range of normal weights. Or simply take 5% to 10% of her current weight as the first goal. If she is very obese (e.g., >99th percentile), the intermediate goals could be stepwise moves to moderately obese, then mildly obese, then overweight, and then normal. This will take time. If she is very obese, you and she should discuss this with her physician, as other options are available, such as medication or even surgery (see Questions 69–79 and Question 82).

Try the ideal body weight calculator at: http://pediatrics. about.com/cs/growthcharts2/l/bl_ibw_calc.htm. Put in her current height and weight, and you will be given her percentile and category (normal, overweight, obese) and the number of pounds needed to reach the top of the normal percentile (85%). Better yet, speak with your daughter's physician to work out a strategy for weight control. This may involve working with a nutritionist or dietitian and perhaps joining a support group.

44. What is involved in the weight-loss program for our daughter? Just a diet?

A good weight-reduction program that will work and will keep the weight off has three components:

- Diet
- Exercise
- Behavioral changes

We will talk about each of these in detail.

Unfortunately, there is no magic solution. If your daughter is overweight or obese and is prone to remain so, then staying at a healthy weight will be a constant battle. The body uses various mechanisms to maintain a stable weight, and if that weight is high, the mechanisms fight to keep the excess weight.

Losing weight will require a lifestyle change and a move away from the typical diet of many American children and teenagers: irregular eating habits and times, lots of fast-food, sugary drinks, high-fat and unbalanced meals, and unhealthy snacking. This will be very hard since people like high-fat fast-foods and sugary drinks.

There must be a change in these three components. The first component, diet, will require regular meals and snacks. A diet must be chosen (there are many) and followed. This will mean limiting portion size and certain foods. The second, exercise, will help use up more calories, speeding weight loss. In a well-designed exercise program, there will be a build up of muscles. This also aids in weight loss, as more muscles use up more energy. The last, and perhaps the hardest, is an attitude and behavior change. There are various techniques to do this and they will be discussed. To remain thin and healthy, your daughter will need to develop a new lifestyle in terms of eating and exercising. This will not be a 4-week or even a 4-month diet but a life-long way of living.

45. What do we have to do for our daughter to lose 1 to 2 pounds per week?

First, let's talk about calories. We need to discuss what calories are, how many your daughter uses each day, and where calories come from.

A calorie is a unit of energy. Calories are consumed in food or beverages that contain proteins, carbohydrates, and fats. The basic rules are simple. Your daughter will gain weight if she consumes more calories per day than she burns. She will lose weight if she burns more calories than she consumes. And of course, her weight will not change if calories in equals calories out. One pound equals 3,500 calories. So, if she eats 3,500 more calories than she uses, she will gain a pound, and if she uses 3,500 more calories than she consumes, she will lose a pound.

One gram (about 1/454 of a pound or 0.03 ounce) of protein or carbohydrate has four calories, and one gram of fat has nine calories. Thus, she will gain more weight per gram of food eaten if she eats fat rather than carbohydrates and proteins. The next steps are to see how many calories are used each day in various activities and then how many calories there are in different types of foods.

46. How many calories does my daughter use each day?

You use calories by simply being alive! Breathing, moving, having your heart beat, etc. use calories. Even while sleeping, you use calories. Here are some examples. Note that the calories used are approximate because they vary by weight—the heavier a person is, the more calories used.

The more physical activity one does, the more calories that person uses. For example, sleeping uses about 60 calories an hour and sitting about 120 calories an hour. The following are calories used for various low-level activities for a person weighing about 150 pounds:

- Bed rest and sleeping, 60 per hour
- Showering (one-fourth hour), 65 cal
- Sitting and thinking, 120 per hour

Table 5 shows calories used for various moderate-to-vigorous level activities for a person weighing 154 pounds.

(See Resources for online calculators for calories per activity by body weight, age, and gender.)

Table 5   The calories burned through physical activity (154 lb, 5'10" tall man).

Moderate Physical Activities	Approximate Calories Used	
	In 1 Hour	In 30 Minutes
Hiking	370	185
Light gardening/yard work	330	165
Dancing	330	165
Golf (walking and carrying club)	330	165
Bicycling (less than 10 miles per hour)	290	145
Walking (3 1/2 miles per hour)	280	140
Weight training (general light workout)	220	110
Stretching	180	90
Vigorous Physical Activities	**In 1 Hour**	**In 30 Minutes**
Running/jogging (5 miles per hour)	590	295
Bicycling (more than 10 miles per hour)	590	295
Swimming (slow freestyle laps)	510	255
Aerobics	480	240
Walking (4 1/2 miles per hour)	460	230
Heavy yard work (chopping wood)	440	220
Weight lifting (vigorous effort)	440	220
Basketball (vigorous)	440	220

United States Department of Agriculture.

The amount of calories used per day depends on many factors, including age, gender, weight, and, of course, the amount of activity done.

47. Assuming that my daughter does some combination of these activities, how many calories per day does she use?

The amount of calories used per day depends on many factors, including age, gender, weight, and, of course, the amount of activity done. Various tables and calculators will give you an approximate number of calories burned per day. They are listed at the end of this section.

The calories needed and used each day can be divided into three groups:

1. **Basal metabolic rate**: This is the energy the body uses to stay alive: keeping the heart pumping, the blood circulating, and so forth. For nonathletes, this takes about 50% to 75% of the total calories used per day. The number of calories used for the basal metabolic rate can be estimated easily by taking your daughter's weight in pounds and multiplying by 10. If she weighs 120, then she will use about $120 \times 10 = 1{,}200$ calories. For a male, the number is slightly higher—pounds $\times$ 11. For your son at 145 pounds, he would use about $145 \times 11 = 1{,}595$ calories a day for basal metabolism.

2. Thermal effect of food: The body uses energy to metabolize and use the food eaten each day. This depends on the number of calories eaten and is approximately 10% of the day's calories. So if your daughter eats 2,500 calories per day, she uses about 250 of them to digest and use the food and drink consumed.

3. Daily activities: This varies depending on how active your child is. A child who never sits down and is always doing something uses more calories than the one who is sitting all day.

This can be complex to calculate if you want to get an exact figure. You'd need to determine how many hours your daughter sleeps, sits, walks, exercises, and so forth. But if you want a quick rule of thumb, this formula comes close. Decide which of the following categories your daughter falls under:

- Light activity (300 calories): Not much movement—mainly sitting, reading, and driving.

Basal metabolic rate

The minimum energy needed or used by the body at complete rest to stay alive (keeping the heart pumping, breathing, blood circulating, and so forth).

- Moderate activity (500 calories): Moving about during the day with lots of walking and some physical activity.
- Heavy activity (700 calories): Moves about a lot during the day and does a lot of sports or other heavy duty activities.

Then use this quick formula to figure out how many calories a day she uses to maintain her current weight. For your daughter, who does light activity and weighs 120 pounds,

$$120 \times 10 = 1,200 + 300 = 1,500 \text{ calories a day}$$

For your son, who does moderate activity and weighs 145 pounds,

$$145 \times 11 = 1,595 + 500 = 2,095 \text{ calories a day}$$

You can make more precise calculations using the table or one of these websites, but the rough calculation should work well. You can also consult your daughter's nutritionist. Don't be concerned if the results differ a bit in each calculator. They are all estimates:

www.diet-blog.com/archives/2005/12/26/how_to_calculate_your_daily_calorie_needs.php

http://calculators-free.com/bmr-and-daily-calories-burned-calculator-9

http://health.drgily.com/basal-metabolic-rate-calculator.php

http://caloriecount.about.com/cc/calories-burned.php

http://walking.about.com/cs/calories/l/blcalcalc.htm

These calculators are more complex and require estimating hours doing certain activities:

www.stevenscreek.com/goodies/calories.shtml

www.preventdisease.com/healthtools/articles/bmr.html

You will see that the calculators give somewhat different results; estimating activity levels is not an exact science.

48. We calculate that our daughter uses 1,500 calories a day. How do we arrange this so that she loses a pound or two a week?

As noted earlier, there are 3,500 calories in a pound. If she wishes to lose 1 pound per week, your daughter needs to use 3,500 more calories a week than she eats. This means 3,500 calories/7 days = 500 calories less a day, making a daily intake of 1,000 calories a day. For your son, this would be 2,095 calories minus 500 = 1,595 calories a day.

This sounds like a significant drop in calories, especially for your daughter who is starting about 500 calories lower than your son, as her weight is less. Dieting is not easy, however, and the numbers cannot be fudged.

There are two ways to influence weight loss: eat fewer calories and increase daily activity. Thus, the way to avoid such a drastic drop in food eaten per day is to increase activity and exercise. This is discussed in Question 49.

Your daughter should not drop below 1,000 calories a day on any diet, as this is not healthy. In addition, interestingly, below 1,000 calories a day the body reacts by slowing the metabolism and thus slowing weight loss, too. The body will also start using muscle for energy. This is not good because it will result in a loss of muscle mass.

If your daughter is at a stable weight now, she is consuming 1,500 calories a day. If she is gaining weight, then she is eating more than 1,500 calories a day. Stay at the current activity level but eat 500 fewer calories a day, or increase the physical activity so that she can eat more each day.

49. How do we set the balance for less food and more activity and exercise?

If your daughter wants to drop 500 calories a day, she can either eat 500 fewer calories each day, increase her activity and exercise by 500 calories a day, or use some combination of the two. First, she needs to do a calorie inventory. If she's already seeing a doctor or a nutritionist, then perhaps this diary was already completed. If not, now is the time to do one. It is easy to do. For 3 days or so, your daughter should carry a little notebook or memo pad and write down everything that she consumes. These should be normal and typical days—not when she is sick or doing something special. She should date the top of the page and write these items:

- Write down everything she eats and drinks, including portion size or weight (e.g., 12 ounces of Diet Coke or a Big Mac with Cheese and a small fries or a turkey wrap with two slices of turkey, lettuce, and tomato with mayonnaise and a 1-ounce bag of potato chips). If she is not sure, estimate.
- If possible, record the calories. They are listed on the label of purchased foods. If not, we will calculate calories later. (See Question 51 about food labels.)
- Include snacks and "grazing" (eating a bit here and there while on the run), drinks, tastes, and so forth.
- Note the time (and place if desired).

Treatment

At the end of the 3 days, put the foods eaten into a list or table, and add up the calories. You can create a table by hand or on your computer. Many websites also have free food diaries or tell you how to keep one by hand (see Resources for some examples). You can search online for "food diary," and you will find many.

Record the calories listed on the food package, or, if you don't have packaging, look in a calorie book or online. In Table 6, the calorie numbers with an asterisk were taken directly from the package, and the ones

Table 6   Example of a calorie inventory.

Date/Time	Food or Drink	How Much	Notes	Calories
January 23 at 7:00 a.m.	Orange juice, not sweetened	6 ounces	Breakfast	80
7:00 a.m.	Rice Krispies	1 cup	Breakfast	100*
7:00 a.m.	Whole milk	0.5 cup	Breakfast	150*
11:00 a.m.	Snickers bar	2 ounces	Snack	273*
11:30 a.m.	Pepsi	12-ounce can	Snack	150*
1:00 p.m.	White bread Ham Mustard Lettuce	2 slices 3 slices 1 teaspoon 2 leaves	Lunch Ham sandwich	135 140 5
1:00 p.m.	Pepsi	12-ounce can	Lunch	150*
1:00 p.m.	Lays potato chips	1-ounce bag	Lunch	150*
2:00 p.m.	Chocolate chip cookie	Small (1 oz?)	Snack	50
7:00 p.m.	Big Mac	1	Dinner	576
7:00 p.m.	Medium fries	1	Dinner	380
7:00 p.m.	Chocolate shake from McDonalds	15 ounces	Dinner	580
10 p.m.	Apple	1 medium	Snack	65
Total				2,984

without were found online or in a book. Online sources include the following:

http://www.calorieking.com

http://caloriecount.about.com

http://www.thecaloriecounter.com

You can simply Google the words "calorie" and the food in question (e.g., "lettuce"). You can find a book at the library or buy an inexpensive book with lists of foods (including fast-foods) (e.g., *2009 CalorieKing Calorie, Fat and Carbohydrate Counter* by Allan Borushek). Do not worry if the different books or databases vary a bit. They are all pretty close. Now take the total calories consumed for the day. For the previous chart, it is 2,984 calories, which is rather high. As you can see, dinner was the big-calorie meal.

Do this for each day, and then analyze the results as described in the next question.

50. Now that I have the charts, how do we analyze them?

Let us analyze Table 6. First, we will start with the total calories. Using the previous example and knowing that your daughter's calorie intake is 1,500 calories per day to maintain her current weight, we see, at least from the previous table, that she is well above her maintenance intake. At this rate, she will gain weight—and fairly quickly.

Let us look at the different parts of the table.

- Did she eat three meals? Yes. Did she have meals and snacks regularly and frequently? Yes, although there was a 5-hour gap between the 2 p.m. snack and the 7 p.m. dinner. More about timing is discussed later.

- Was the calorie distribution balanced? In this case, no. Dinner accounted for about one-half of the day's calories.
- What did she eat? Was it balanced? We will talk more about balance and food groups later, but just looking quickly at this table, we see lots of sugary drinks, only one fruit, and minimal vegetables (lettuce and tomato on the ham sandwich and whatever was in the Big Mac). There were a lot of carbohydrates (OJ, bread, Snickers, Pepsis, shake, fries, cookie, chips), some fat and protein (Big Mac, fries, ham) and almost no fiber (apple, lettuce, tomato). This was a heavy-carbohydrate day.
- How was the food prepared? Was there a lot of fried food? Was there healthier baked, grilled, or steamed food?

There were too many calories, too many carbohydrates, too many sugary drinks, not much fiber and the meals were not well balanced.

51. I've seen the food labels on the packages of food I buy. How do I analyze them?

The U.S. government requires that food labels are placed on products sold to the public, and specific regulations must be followed. This is a good time to look at a food label and analyze its components. Here are two food labels. The first is for a Big Mac (Figure 1).

The second is for an apple (Figure 2).

You can find labels scalable by portion size for a variety of foods at: www.caloriecount.about.com/foods and at: www.nutritiondata.com. In addition, the Food and Drug Administration (FDA) has a good website

The U.S. government requires that food labels are placed on products sold to the public, and specific regulations must be followed.

Nutrition Facts

Serving Size 1 sandwich (215.0 g)

Amount Per Serving

Calories 576	Calories from Fat 292

% Daily Value*

Total Fat 32.5g	**50%**
Saturated Fat 12.0g	**60%**
Polyunsaturated Fat 2.8g	
Monounsaturated Fat 14.1g	
Cholesterol 103mg	**34%**
Sodium 742mg	**31%**
Total Carbohydrates 38.7g	**13%**
Protein 31.8g	

Vitamin A 1%	•	Vitamin C 2%
Calcium 9%	•	Iron 31%

* Based on a 2000 calorie diet

BIG MAC

- ← 1. Size Portion
- ← 2. Total calories & fat calories
- ← 3. Fat
- ← 4. Cholesterol
- ← 5. Sodium (salt)
- ← 6. Carbohydrates
- ← 7. Protein
- ← 8. Vitamins & minerals

Figure 1   Food Label for a Big Mac Hamburger

Nutrition Facts

Serving Size
1 large (3 1/4" diameter) (approx. 2 per lb)

Amount Per Serving

Calories 110	Calories from Fat 3

% Daily Value*

Total Fat 0.4g	**1%**
Saturated Fat 0.1g	**0%**
Polyunsaturated Fat 0.1g	
Monounsaturated Fat 0.0g	
Cholesterol 0mg	**0%**
Sodium 2mg	**0%**
Total Carbohydrates 29.3g	**10%**
Dietary Fiber 5.1g	**20%**
Sugars 22.0g	
Protein 0.6g	

Vitamin A 2%	•	Vitamin C 16%
Calcium 1%	•	Iron 1%

* Based on a 2000 calorie diet

APPLE

- ← 1. Size Portion
- ← 2. Total calories & fat calories
- ← 3. Fat
- ← 4. Cholesterol
- ← 5. Sodium (salt)
- ← 6. Carbohydrates
- ← 7. Protein
- ← 8. Vitamins & minerals

Figure 2   Food Label for an Apple

devoted to reading a food label: www.cfsan.fda.gov/~dms/foodlab.html.

Let's look at what these labels say. The first line identifies the product. For the Big Mac, we see that it is a sandwich and that the serving size is 1 sandwich, which weighs 215 grams. Some of the labels are in grams (metric), some in ounces (American system), and sometimes both. There are 454 grams in a pound (16 ounces). Thus, 215 grams is a bit less than half a pound (about 7.5 ounces). One gram then is about 1/450 of a pound or about 1/30 of an ounce—that is very small.

Sometimes the labels are not written in a user-friendly way. For example, a container of dark chocolate fudge brownie mix weighs 1 pound and 3.9 ounces. Each serving size is 1/20 of the package, and there are 20 servings per package. Each serving before making the brownies has 110 calories, and each serving after making the brownies has 170 calories. It is very hard to know how many calories are in a single brownie unless you cut the whole pan of brownies into 20 equal pieces.

Line 2 shows the number of calories in a serving and the number of these calories that are from fat. For the Big Mac, there are 576 calories, of which over half are from fat. The apple has 110 calories, of which 3 are from fat and the remaining calories from carbohydrates (simple sugars, 22 grams or 88 calories; complex sugars, about 2 or 3 grams or 8 to 12 calories). The numbers are slightly different from the total because of rounding and approximation. Don't worry about this. Just get a rough feel for the calories.

Line 3 gives more information about the fat. For the sandwich, each serving has 32.5 grams of fat, of which

12 grams are saturated ("bad" fat); 2.8 grams are polyunsaturated ("good" fat); and 14.1 grams are monounsaturated ("not so good" fat); The apple has almost no fat, and the little it has is split between saturated and polyunsaturated fat. At 9 calories per gram of fat, you can see the sandwich has 32.5 × 9 or over 290 calories from fat. The apple has only 3 calories from fat.

Line 4 is total cholesterol. Cholesterol is another type of lipid that actually consists of various components, including HDL ("good" cholesterol) and LDL ("bad" cholesterol). The breakdown is not given here, so there is no way to know this information from the label. The Big Mac has 103 mg of cholesterol and the apple none at all.

Obviously, one sandwich is supplying two-thirds of daily fat, one-third of the daily cholesterol, and one-third of daily salt. This is a lot for a single item consumed at one meal and means that the intake for the rest of the day should limit the fat and salt.

Look at the percentage daily value column on the chart. In the examples, these percentages are based on a 2,000-calorie diet. This number of calories may or may not be the actual number that your child consumes now or will consume on a diet. Use them as a rough approximation of required intake. The message here is that the sandwich has a lot of fat, whereas the apple does not. Some of the online tools allow you to calculate the calorie diet to use as the basis of calculating the percentage daily value.

Line 5 is the amount of salt (actually sodium) per serving. The typical American diet probably includes too much salt, especially in prepared foods, and many authorities feel that this contributes to high blood pressure and other health problems. The sandwich has 742 mg of sodium, which is about one-third of the daily intake. Unlike calories, the amount of minerals and vitamins a person needs really does not differ very much by his or her weight. Thus, the daily percentage of sodium listed here is applicable to just about everyone whether at a healthy weight or not. The sandwich has a lot of salt and the apple almost none (2 mg).

Line 6 shows the carbohydrates, including sugars, starches, and some fiber (see Question 53 for much more about carbohydrates). Here is what we can say now: the label lists *total* carbohydrates, which covers so-called simple sugars (such as glucose, fructose, sucrose [table sugar]), fiber (which is not metabolized or digested and passes out through the body without supplying any calories), and complex sugars or starches. These complex carbohydrates are included in the total carbohydrates but are usually not explicitly stated in the breakout section where each carbohydrate is listed. It is not clear why this is not listed. The Big Mac label gives only the total carbohydrates (38.7 grams), whereas the apple label notes 29.3 grams, of which 5.1 grams are fiber and 22 grams are sugars. The remaining carbohydrates, obtained by subtraction (29.3 − 5.1 − 22.0 = 2.2 grams), are complex carbohydrates, such as starches and other "long-chain" molecules. For the apple, the total number of carbohydrates minus the fiber is 24.1 grams, of which the largest part is simple sugar. The carbohydrate story is complex and involves the **glycemic index**, the **glycemic load**, and more (see Question 59 for more details).

Line 7 is protein. The Big Mac has almost 32 grams of protein and the apple almost none. As protein has

Glycemic index

A number score given to carbohydrates as a function of how high and how quickly they raise blood sugar and insulin. Scores below 55 are low, meaning that they raise blood sugar slowly; scores above 70 cause a rapid rise in blood sugar.

Glycemic load

A calculation based on the glycemic index multiplied by the number of grams of carbohydrates, all of which is then multiplied by 100. This is an extension of the glycemic index in that it accounts for the amount of carbohydrates eaten and is useful in meal planning.

4 calories per gram, the sandwich would have about 128 calories from protein and the apple none.

Line 8 represents certain key vitamins and minerals. As you can see, neither the apple nor the Big Mac supplies many vitamins and minerals, except for a good amount of iron in the beef in the Big Mac. It is usually a good idea to take a multivitamin/mineral pill while on a weight-loss diet to ensure that all of the needed ones are consumed.

Finally, some labels will have a footnote with recommended daily intakes for certain components of the diet: fat, cholesterol, sodium, carbohydrates, and fiber. Most labels are based on 2,000-calorie (or 2,500-calorie) diets and are too high for your child if she is on a lower calorie diet. In addition, some have criticized the fiber figure as being too low. Many feel at least 35 grams a day of fiber should be consumed (Table 7).

Table 7   Sample of a percent daily values label.

	Calories	2,000	2,500
Total Fat	Less than	65g	80g
Sat Fat	Less than	20g	25g
Cholesterol	Less than	300mg	300mg
Sodium	Less than	2,400mg	2,400mg
Total Carbohydrate		300g	375g
Dietary Fiber		25g	30g

52. I have the charts, the food diary, the number of calories that my daughter should consume each day, and the exercise suggestions to lose weight. What diet should I choose? Thousands of different diet books are available, and each says that it has a revolutionary and guaranteed weight-loss program. Could you review the diets?

Many diets are available. One of them alternates a fasting day with a light eating day. Some revolve around a particular food ("the grapefruit diet" or "the rice diet"). Some rotate different diets. Some are ethnic or regional (e.g., Mediterranean). Others are high fat, whereas others are low fat. Some are liquid only (some of these were deadly—discussed more later). We'll review many of them but begin with the balanced-calorie counting diet based on the Food Pyramid. Then we look at some of the other more mainstream diets and finish with the more gimmicky or outlandish ones.

Weight loss will occur by eating less than you eat now or increasing your exercise or energy expenditures without increasing your calorie intake. It requires effort and some will power. Most of all it requires a commitment to changes in lifestyle. Unless your child is one of those people who can eat all she wants and never gain an ounce (and if she is, you would probably not be reading this book), diet and lifestyle change has to be a lifelong commitment. It requires a change in thinking and outlook and a realization that she is not one of those people who can eat whatever she wants whenever she wants. This is not "fair" but there is no other way. (We will talk more about the psychology of dieting later.)

Whenever you see a diet that uses one or more of the words or phrases below, be very skeptical. There is no magic.

- Revolutionary
- Magic or miraculous
- Guaranteed
- 100% successful
- Miracle diet
- Eat anything you want
- Eat as much as you want
- Eliminates all food cravings
- Suppressed by the medical establishment
- New
- Free
- Lose a lot of weight rapidly (e.g., 12 pounds in 1 week)
- No-fail

Be somewhat skeptical of celebrity endorsements, personal stories, or anecdotes. Most diets followed for a short length of time (weeks) will produce weight loss—though this is often only body water and not body fat.

Be somewhat skeptical of celebrity endorsements, personal stories, or anecdotes. Most diets followed for a short length of time (weeks) will produce weight loss—though this is often only body water and not body fat. Whether the diets are doable over long periods and whether the weight comes back are crucial to know. It would be good to see the celebrities or people giving testimonials a year or two later. In the occasional case when we do, such as with Oprah Winfrey, we see that she has lost a large amount of weight but regained it over time. She has "yo-yoed" between about 160 and 237 pounds using a variety of diets.

53. What is the Atkins Diet?

Those who support this diet feel that overweight and obese people eat too many carbohydrates, particularly refined carbohydrates such as simple sugars, white rice, milk, white flour products (pasta), and other "bad" carbohydrates. First, some information on carbohydrates. Carbohydrates are rapidly absorbed into the bloodstream. The body, sensing a carbohydrate load, then secretes the hormone insulin from the pancreas. Insulin then causes the sugar to be converted into a more complex sugar called **glycogen**, which is stored in the liver and in muscles. This storage capacity is rather limited in the body, however, and the sugar that cannot be stored is then converted by insulin into fat and stored in the body around the abdomen (the belly), the thighs, the hips/buttocks, and elsewhere.

Glycogen

A complex sugar (carbohydrate) that the body makes from many glucose molecules chained together. It is used to store energy for later use.

Insulin must be secreted frequently during the day to deal with the carbohydrate loads from meals and snacks. Over time, this causes the body to become less sensitive to insulin ("insulin insensitivity") and leads to large swings in blood sugar ("unstable blood sugar") and ultimately to diabetes.

To combat this vicious cycle, the Atkins Diet requires that fat and protein, rather than carbohydrates, become the main components of the diet. By doing this, the body moves into a metabolic state called **ketosis**. Ketosis represents the increase in the body of ketones (also called ketone bodies)—chemicals that are the products of the metabolism of fats. Carbohydrate metabolism does not produce ketones or ketosis. The proponents of this type of diet claim that the chronic ketosis is not harmful and produces various beneficial things such as the burning of the fat—both ingested as well as stored fat producing weight loss. The ketosis also decreases the appetite (it is claimed) and will ultimately lead away from insulin insensitivity, diabetes, and a return to normal metabolism. Actually, blood fat levels in some

Ketosis

An increase of ketones (also called ketone bodies) in the blood. Ketones are chemicals produced by the body from the normal metabolism of fat. For long periods, however, high ketone levels can cause certain problems, particularly in the kidney and liver.

cases will ultimately decrease (even though you are eating a high-fat diet) after an initial spike.

For many years, the medical establishment did not recognize this concept (which dates back to the 19th century), but now, with new data, particularly from clinical trials, there is some grudging acceptance that there really is something to this idea. More work still needs to be done. The long-term effects of high-fat/high-protein and low-carbohydrate diets are unknown. We will surely hear more about this over the coming years.

54. What are the specifics of the Atkins Diet?

The idea is to limit one's carbohydrate intake to 20 grams a day during the first 2 weeks of the diet (the "induction phase") and then increase it to 40 grams a day. This is the level at which the body changes its metabolism to produce ketosis. Exercise is good to help induce ketosis and burn fat. Because this is not a balanced diet (little fruit, only certain vegetables), a multiple vitamin/mineral pill should also be taken each day.

After the 2-week induction phase is over and the body has moved into its new ketosis state, a small amount of good carbohydrates (whole-grain products and some fruits and vegetables) can be added, bringing the total up to 40 grams a day. This is actually a very small amount (about 160 calories). The bad carbohydrates (pasta, white rice, milk, white bread, and potatoes—anything made from refined sugar or white flour) must be avoided basically forever.

Many kinds of fats can be eaten (butter, milk, mayonnaise, etc.), although trans fats (partially hydrogenated oils) should be avoided. These are commonly found in fried foods and fast-foods such as donuts, fried potatoes, pastry, pies, cookies, and stick margarine. A tendency now exists in the United States to substitute less harmful fats for trans fats, and many communities have passed local laws requiring restaurants to avoid using trans fats. In a sense, calories do not count, although some feel that the ketosis decreases the appetite and leads to a lower calorie intake. Some people become accustomed to the ketosis and are able to eat a high-calorie diet, leading to a cessation of weight loss or even weight gain. No matter what diet is used, the bottom line is that calories taken must be lower than calories expended for you to lose weight.

No matter what diet is used, the bottom line is that calories taken must be lower than calories expended for you to lose weight.

As you move into the maintenance phase, good carbohydrates can slowly be added until weight loss stops. This then determines how many carbohydrates you can eat per day without regaining the weight that has been lost. The number of allowed carbohydrates per day varies from person to person but is usually about 40 grams per day.

55. Does Atkins work? What are the up sides?

Yes, the Atkins Diet clearly works for some people. Quick weight loss occurs, especially during the first several weeks. Some people are able to tolerate the ketosis for long periods and lose a lot of weight; however, as soon as you start eating more carbohydrates (even if you do not eat them at the previous level), much or all of the weight rapidly returns.

The medical establishment was largely skeptical of the diet for many years but has now conceded that weight loss is possible if the diet is followed. Some maintain that it is simply another way to decrease calorie intake and that this diet, like any diet where you use more calories than you take in, will lead to weight loss—whether

Treatment

the calories are in the form of a balanced diet, all fat/protein, or three chocolate shakes a day (and nothing else). Because it is very hard, if not impossible, to accurately track and measure calories ingested per day over long periods, it is very difficult to prove or refute the idea that fewer calories are ingested. Some Atkins advocates claim that more calories can be ingested per day with weight loss on this diet compared with other diets because of the change in metabolism.

56. What are the possible risks and downsides of the Atkins Diet, particularly in my child?

Several possible downsides exist. The first is the claim that this diet is simply an unbalanced, low-calorie diet in which almost all of the calories come from fats and proteins. Nothing is new or startling here. Yes, there is ketosis, but there is still no "magic" in this diet. Whether diabetes can be prevented remains to be seen. Clearly, by losing weight, insulin sensitivity can return and diabetes controlled or possibly prevented or delayed; however, whether this is due to the lack of carbohydrates in the diet or simply the weight loss is unclear. Also, unless you rigorously stick to the diet—a permanent lifestyle change—the weight will come back over time.

Unfortunately, ketosis, for some people, is unpleasant, although not usually dangerous. They may feel light-headed or dizzy and nauseated. In diabetics (who should not follow Atkins without consulting their physician), there is a much more severe related condition called ketoacidosis, which can be a medical emergency. This is different from the ketosis of the low-carbohydrate diet. Also, a high-protein intake may lead to an increase in kidney stones and a decrease in kidney function in some people.

Many authorities feel that the greatest risk with this and other high-fat diets is an increased risk of heart disease, stroke, and certain cancers. For many years, it was felt that a high-fat diet would increase lipid levels in the blood and cause an increase in heart disease and strokes. This is somewhat less clear now, as some evidence shows that the high-fat Atkins Diet can actually lead to lower—not higher—blood lipid levels. Because high blood lipid levels increase the risk and danger of heart disease, the weakening of the link between a high-fat diet and high blood lipids leaves open the question of whether a high-fat diet without increased blood lipid levels can lead to heart disease. Many still feel that it can, but no definitive answer yet exists.

With children, there is even more controversy. On one hand, some authorities feel that the risks associated with obesity in children are so great that any possible dangers the Atkins Diet might have are outweighed if the diet is successful. Such ketogenic diets are used to treat some forms of epilepsy that are resistant to medications, and research is being conducted to test this in children. Others feel that developmentally this diet would be dangerous for children, especially younger children, as they are not getting all of the balanced nutrients needed for good development. There is little to no data about the use of the Atkins Diet in children. And last, we do not have much data on people using the diet for 20, 30, or 40 years both in terms of benefits (keeping the weight off) and risks.

57. Is Atkins controversial and maybe even dangerous?

Yes, the theory and science behind this diet are quite controversial. The idea of high-fat/high-protein, low-carbohydrate diets actually dates back to the 19th century and earlier. For a while, this idea for weight control and diet caught on in the late 1800s and early 1900s.

By the late 20th century, however, the medical community felt that the high-fat diet led to high blood fats (lipids such as cholesterol and triglycerides), which led to heart disease and strokes. The high rates of heart attacks and strokes seemed to be caused by the combination of a high-fat diet, a lack of exercise, and increased calories each day. The high-fat/high-protein diets fell into disrepute, although, as noted, they have been around long before Dr. Atkins repopularized and extended this concept. The medical community is currently reexamining the high-fat/high-protein diets and is doing laboratory and clinical experiments and trials to better understand what is happening, especially because the obesity epidemic is worsening.

Most authorities, including the U.S. government, recommend a "classic" balanced low-calorie diet and lifestyle change.

In adults, where some data exist, the situation is still confusing and controversial. In children, where almost no data are available, there is little valid science available to draw a conclusion. At this point, the benefits, risks, and dangers are unclear. Most authorities, including the U.S. government, recommend a "classic" balanced low-calorie diet and lifestyle change. This is probably the safest and most appropriate course of action to take at this time (see the References at the end of the book for further reading).

58. What about the South Beach Diet and other low-carbohydrate diets?

The South Beach Diet is a low-carbohydrate diet similar to the Atkins Diet. Like the Atkins Diet, it has an induction and then a maintenance period. The South Beach diet refers to the glycemic index, whereas the Atkins Diet refers to the glycemic load (see Question 59), as a way to determine good and bad carbohydrates.

The South Beach Diet avoids saturated fats (e.g., butter) somewhat more than Atkins. Both avoid trans fats. The way that permitted carbohydrates are calculated also varies. Atkins uses carbohydrate counting by grams. That is, except for nonabsorbable carbohydrates, you have to count the number of grams of carbohydrates eaten per day. South Beach uses a slightly different technique, using portion size and the number of carbohydrates eaten.

Multiple variations on the high-fat, low-carbohydrate diets exist (see Resources). Some are quite radical and strange, such as a meat-only diet. There is little or no data on these diets. As noted previously, be very careful about using such a diet for your child. The risks and dangers are not clearly known, especially in children.

59. What is the glycemic index, and what is a glycemic load?

These are related concepts that help in evaluating whether a carbohydrate is "good or bad," that is, whether it has a major effect on blood glucose or not. Because different carbohydrates raise blood sugar in different amounts and at different rates, these measurements were developed to quantify this.

The glycemic index gives a numerical score to carbohydrates as a function of how high and how quickly they raise blood sugar and insulin. Scores below 55 have a low glycemic index, as they raise the levels slowly, which is considered good. Scores above 70 cause blood glucose and insulin to rise quickly, which is considered bad.

Scores between 55 and 70 are intermediate. Many things affect the glycemic index, including the type of sugar/starch in the food; how the food is processed and cooked; and whether fiber, fat, protein, and other components are present. The glycemic index does not account for portion size, however.

The glycemic load uses the glycemic index plus portion size to calculate a value. The formula is as follows:

glycemic load = (glycemic index × grams of carbohydrate)/100

The glycemic index is useful in figuring out substitutions when planning a meal or diet. The glycemic load is useful in calculating how much of something to eat and is used in some of the low-carbohydrate diets to calculate the quantity of certain carbohydrates that are allowed.

Low-carbohydrate diets are by definition low-glycemic-load diets. Some evidence shows that low-glycemic-load diets lower the risk for diabetes and heart disease and possibly obesity and cancer. Low-carbohydrate diets that use glycemic index and/or glycemic load have extensive lists and tables on their calculation and use in preparing meals and choosing foods.

60. What is the Mediterranean diet, and can it be used in children?

The Mediterranean diet mimics the eating habits of the people living in southern Europe and northern Africa/Middle East. There is no one single Mediterranean diet, as 16 different countries with many different groups of people border the Mediterranean Sea.

In general, this diet means eating much fish and little red meat, lots of fruits and vegetables, grain and (nonwhite flour) breads, pasta, rice, "healthy fats" such as olive oil and canola oil, nuts, and sometimes, for adults, moderate amounts of red wine. In this diet, portions are moderate, and little dairy food (some cheese and yogurt are allowed) and few saturated fats (butter) or trans fats are consumed. Junk food, as we know it, is not included.

This diet is similar to the recommendations in the American Heart Association diet, although it contains more fat than the American Heart Association diet recommendations. Nonetheless, this diet is felt to be heart healthy.

Preliminary evidence shows that certain childhood illnesses such as allergies and asthma are less frequent in children on this diet. With small modifications, this diet can easily be adapted for children, especially because some sweets, peanut butter, pasta, and fruits are allowed.

61. What is the anti-inflammatory diet?

Some foods clearly produce disease, allergies, and inflammation. For example, some individuals have **celiac disease**, which is an inflammatory disease of the small intestine caused by eating products containing gluten (found mainly in grains such as wheat, barley, or rye). Removal of gluten from the diet results in improvement of the disease in most cases. Similarly, up to 8% of babies and young children may have an allergy to various food products such as fish, shellfish, peanuts and other nuts, eggs, and milk. Interestingly, chocolate is a rare food allergy. Treatment in most cases involves determining the offending foods and removing them from the diet.

By extension, various diets have been proposed that seem to decrease inflammation, not just due to certain well-known offending foods, as noted previously, but to

Celiac disease

A disease of the small intestine in which gluten containing foods are not tolerated producing diarrhea and other gastrointestinal symptoms. It is also called "nontropical sprue" or "gluten intolerance."

many other foods, including junk foods, trans and saturated fats, refined sugar, and meat. "Anti-inflammatory" diets instruct you to avoid these items in the hope that various diseases due to inflammation such as asthma and arthritis will be improved or prevented. In addition, certain drugs or other products such as omega-3 fatty acids (found in fish oil, walnuts, and canola oil) and olive oil are recommended as anti-inflammatory agents. Although there is not a lot of data in support of them, these diets certainly seem to do no harm. In fact, the anti-inflammatory diet resembles a well-balanced reducing diet or the Mediterranean diet. We have come to the same conclusion via a different route. This diet is fine for your child.

62. What is a low-fat diet? Does it differ from the other diets?

Various sorts of low fat diets are proposed for reducing weight, lowering blood lipids (high cholesterol, high triglycerides), treating certain diseases (e.g., gallstones, pancreatic malabsorption problems, and fatty liver), or simply for providing "good health." These diets avoid fatty foods, fried foods, many dairy foods, junk foods, red meat, butter, and most oils. In particular, they try to avoid saturated and trans fats, which have been implicated in heart disease and strokes. Trans fats are mainly vegetable oils to which hydrogen has been added chemically ("hydrogenation") to stiffen or "solidify" the fat. The resulting fats are used in processed foods such as cookies, crackers, potato chips, margarine, and other foods. Saturated fats are also hydrogenated but are found more commonly in animal fats. Beef, lamb, pork, lard, cream, butter, and cheese all have saturated fats. These foods also have cholesterol. Some plant fats such as palm oil and coconut oil also contain saturated fats but no cholesterol.

Obviously, a low-fat diet differs from the Atkins and South Beach high-fat/high-protein diets. It is more like the well-balanced reducing diet or the Mediterranean diet. This too is fine for your child.

63. What are the single-food diets (such as the rice diet or the grapefruit diet) and liquid diets?

There have been many so-called single-food diets over the years. Actually, they weren't really single-food diets in most cases but rather a diet built around a particular food that appeared to have some sort of special power or an ingredient that produced weight loss.

The grapefruit diet dates back to the 1930s and was also called the Hollywood Diet. It actually was a low-calorie (about 1,000 to 1,200 calories), low-carbohydrate, moderate-fat, and moderate-protein diet with grapefruit. It was recommended for about 2 weeks, and a 10-pound weight loss was claimed. Exercise was also recommended. It generally worked, although it was somewhat repetitive and boring—hence, the recommendation for only 2 weeks at a time. This diet is okay for a short-term weight loss, unless your child is also taking certain drugs that grapefruit juice interferes with, including statins (e.g., Zocor, Lipitor), Saquinivir (an HIV drug), calcium channel blockers (e.g., Procardia), antidepressants (e.g., Buspar or Zoloft), anti-seizure medications such as carbamazepine, heart drugs such as amiodarone, and some **immunosuppressants** (cyclosporine). If your child is taking one of these drugs, talk to your doctor about drug interactions with grapefruit and certain other citrus fruits such as pomelos and Seville oranges. While this is a good short-term diet, the weight will likely return unless your

Immunosuppressants

Drugs that are given to suppress one or more parts of the immune system. They are used to treat many diseases caused by inflammation as well as to prevent transplanted organ rejection.

child makes a change in lifestyle and avoids reverting to prediet eating habits.

Some single-food or "special" diets are actually harmful.

Some single-food or "special" diets are actually harmful. There are many: the egg and tomato diet, the cabbage soup diet, the potato-only diet, and the rice diet. These diets are boring, difficult to maintain for any extended period, unbalanced, and dangerous. They should be avoided.

You may also have heard of liquid diets. There is a place in the medical treatment of certain intestinal diseases (e.g., pancreatic disease, small bowel inflammation, and malabsorption) where a physician will put a patient on a liquid diet for a time. They are also used as part of the "preps" for certain procedures such as colonoscopy; however, for routine weight loss, liquid diets should be avoided. Some were found to actually be harmful and were withdrawn from the market. Check with a physician before contemplating beginning any liquid-only diet.

64. Are vegetarian diets okay?

Vegetarian diets, when managed correctly, are fine. Several types of vegetarian diets exist, ranging from vegan (plant-based food only) to those that use selected nonplant foods such as eggs, milk, cheese, and even fish (avoiding meat only). The key is to get all of the nutrients that your body needs (e.g., protein, carbohydrates, fats, vitamins, minerals such as calcium, and zinc). The more restrictive the diet, the harder it is to ensure that your child is getting everything that she needs. By limiting calories, a vegetarian diet is, of course, a fine way to lose weight. Speak with a dietitian or nutritionist to design a diet that ensures that all needed nutrients are present.

65. Are very low-calorie diets or starvation diets okay?

No, these are not recommended. Low-calorie diets are about 1,000 to 1,600 calories per day. Very low-calorie diets are less than 800 calories per day and are not recommended. Although there is a greater initial weight loss with a very low-calorie diet, studies have shown that at 1 year, low-calorie diets are just as good because much of the very low-calorie diet weight loss is gained back. In addition, nutritional deficiencies can occur on a very low-calorie diet, and you must be sure that multivitamins, minerals, and any other essential nutrients are taken. Some authorities also feel that the very low-calorie diets do not assist in changing long-term behavior and lifestyles because the person knows that he or she will return to a more normal diet at some point. Some people on very a low-calorie diet have an increased incidence of gallstones.

66. Are there scientific studies that compare different diets?

Yes, many studies have been done over the years, but they are very difficult to do for many reasons:

- Large numbers of subjects are needed to get meaningful results.
- The study has to run a long time to see whether the weight is lost and then if it stays off.
- People cannot be hospitalized or institutionalized for long periods to track carefully what they eat.
- It is very hard to control someone's diet if he or she eats outside of the home (e.g., at work or restaurants).
- Keeping a food and drink diary with exact measurements and calorie counts is difficult to do.
- It is hard to measure physical activity.

- The studies cannot be "blinded." That is, the gold standard for medical studies includes double-blinded clinical trials. This means that neither the patients nor the physicians doing the study know which group is getting which treatment. This minimizes bias. It is not feasible or possible to blind a food study.
- Sometimes people "cheat" or exaggerate what they eat or how much they exercise.
- People drop out, move, quit the study, or miss appointments.

Various studies over the years have looked at diets. Most are in adults rather than children, and most run for short lengths of time. We summarize here one well-done study published in the *New England Journal of Medicine* on July 17, 2008, entitled "Weight Loss with a Low-Carbohydrate, Mediterranean, or Low-Fat Diet" by Iris Shai, RD, PhD, and collaborators. This was a 2-year study in which 322 obese adults were randomly assigned to one of three diets:

- Low-fat, restricted calorie
- Mediterranean, restricted calorie
- Low-carbohydrate, nonrestricted calorie

Although there was tight follow-up, 50 of the patients were lost to the study by 2 years (the end of the study). The average weight loss was 6.4 pounds for the low-fat group, 9.7 pounds for the Mediterranean-diet group, and 10.3 pounds for the low-carbohydrate group. Cholesterol levels improved in the low-carbohydrate and low-fat groups. Thirty-six subjects had diabetes. Of these subjects, the glucose and insulin levels changed more favorably in those on the Mediterranean diet. The conclusions here are that at 2 years the best weight loss was about 10 pounds, that all the diets worked—some better than others—and that cholesterol levels improved in both the high-fat (low-carbohydrate) and low-fat groups. For the diabetic subjects, the Mediterranean diet seemed to be the best in terms of glucose and insulin control. Weight loss was maximal at about 5 or 6 months; weight then slowly rose in the low-carbohydrate and low-fat groups by the end of year 2. The Mediterranean diet subjects regained the least weight by 2 years.

Thus, all of the diets seem to work to one degree or another. The peak weight loss occurs early, and some of the weight is regained over time. The big surprise is that serum cholesterol/lipids improved on both the high-fat and low-fat diets.

67. So what is the bottom line on my child's diet? Which one is best?

The U.S. government and the medical authorities recommend the diet that is based on the food pyramid. Check the website at: www.mypyramid.gov. It is based on the government's Dietary Guidelines for Americans. It emphasizes fruits, vegetables, whole grains, and fat-free or low-fat milk and milk products and includes lean meats, poultry, fish, beans, eggs, and nuts and is low in saturated fats, trans fats, cholesterol, salt (sodium), and added sugars. As used here it is a balanced, low-fat, calorie-restricted diet. The website is excellent and has sections for using the diet in preschoolers and 5 to 11 year olds as well as the general public. You should go through the "Steps to a Healthier Weight" screens on this website which let you figure out what to eat, how much to eat, which foods are "nutrient dense" (full of good nutrients but lacking in "empty" calories. There is also an excellent menu planner and diet customizer. These are interactive and let you run various "what if" scenarios. The resources at this site are complex and to set up a good, detailed diet that is really doable for your child, you may want to use this website as a start and then speak with a dietician or nutritionist to help design a practical, detailed diet that is customized for your child and, as emphasized many times in this book, doable and feasible in the real world. That is, the diet would be different for a child who eats out a lot compared to a child who takes most of his or her meals at home.

As an alternative, the Mediterranean diet, with calorie restriction, is only slightly different and is also effective. All diets require careful attention and tracking of what is eaten, and all would be good over long periods. The high-fat/high-protein Atkins-type diets are more controversial, although they are considered more seriously now for some people. Because there is little to no experience in children, it is not possible to recommend this diet for weight loss in children.

The bottom line is that your child (as in adults) has to move to a new lifestyle of healthy eating with less fast-food, less "bad" fat, more exercise, and a balanced diet if weight loss is to be achieved and maintained. It must be a diet that is not dull and that can be kept up over one's lifetime. This can be a tall order, but there is no other way.

68. What about exercise? I understand what you said about doing more exercise to burn calories, but doesn't exercise increase appetite?

Exercise and physical activity are definitely healthy (unless your doctor says not to do so because of a particular disease or condition). It seems to promote good health in many, if not most, of the body's organs: the heart, the muscles, the joints, the intestines, the lungs, and so forth. Specifically, evidence shows that it reduces the risk of hypertension, sudden death, diabetes, colon cancer, back pain, high blood lipids, heart disease, and stroke. Similarly, in people who already have diabetes, heart disease, hypertension, and other diseases, exercise may improve these conditions. Obviously, if there are medical issues, your child's physician should examine any exercise regimen.

There is some controversy regarding exercise and weight loss. Some claim that exercise, while burning calories, actually stimulates the appetite and the net effect is to increase food intake. That is, exercise makes us hungry, and exercise, although generally fine, is not necessarily a component of a successful weight-loss program. Obesity is due more to fat accumulation influenced primarily by one's genetic makeup and by eating too many carbohydrates.

On the other hand, an extensive review by the Cochrane Collaboration looked at 43 studies of over 3,400 subjects. They found that diet with exercise resulted in greater weight loss than diet alone. The more one exercises, the more weight is lost. The Cochrane Collaboration is a highly esteemed medical organization dedicated to evidence-based medicine. They typically review the medical literature and make medical recommendations based only on data and evidence—not on theory, anecdotes, and suppositions.

Another claim for exercise is that it helps build muscle mass. The more muscle a person has the more calories will be burned in any particular activity compared with someone with less muscle. This helps in weight loss.

Currently, the best evidence shows that exercise is indeed good and helps in weight loss.

69. What about medication for weight loss? Some FDA-approved drugs are on the market. Can my child take one of those to make the weight loss easier?

Several drugs may assist in weight loss, but remember—no "magic bullet" exists that makes weight loss rapid and painless.

Several drugs may assist in weight loss, but remember—no "magic bullet" exists that makes weight loss rapid and painless. There are drugs on the market (both prescription and **over the counter**) that can work in addition to a diet and exercise.

Over the counter

A term used to describe drugs legally sold in the United States without a doctor's prescription.

The FDA has not approved any of these drugs for use in children. Thus, they should not be used in children unless it is for significant (or morbid) obesity and is absolutely under the care of a physician with experience in using these drugs in children. You and your child must understand the risks that are involved, and you will all have to pay close attention for any possible side effects or problems that might occur.

70. Many over-the-counter weight-loss products are available. Are they okay? Do I need to have my child see a doctor to use them?

This is a complex area because the laws governing these products in the United States are complicated. Many diet products are not regulated. They fall into a special category that Congress established in 1994 called the Dietary Supplement Health and Education Act (DSHEA). This law changed how the FDA handles weight-loss products. It created two types of products.

The first are products to treat obesity and are not dietary supplements. These are handled like drugs and require FDA review and approval before marketing, and so are considered generally safe and effective. That is, the benefits outweigh the risks when used according to directions in the approved patient group listed in the labeling.

The second type of product includes dietary supplements for weight control or appetite suppression. They are not "drugs." The FDA does not approve these before marketing, but rather looks at only some of them and only after they have been on the market. The FDA does not certify that they are "safe and effective." There is no requirement for clinical studies before marketing, and the manufacturer, not the FDA, determines the dose (serving size) and amount of the dietary supplement. Manufacturers are not required to disclose to the FDA or consumers the information that they have about the safety or purported benefits of their dietary supplement products. The FDA does not routinely monitor or analyze the contents of the products. The manufacturer may not market a dietary supplement product as a treatment or cure for a specific disease or condition. These dietary supplements can contain one or more of the following: vitamins, minerals, herbs or other botanicals, amino acids, enzymes or tissues from organs or glands, concentrates, metabolites, constituents, or extracts. Certain new dietary ingredients must be sent to the FDA, and the manufacturer must show that the new ingredient is "reasonably expected to be safe for use in a dietary supplement, unless it has been recognized as a food substance and is present in the food supply."

Generally, the FDA gets involved only if there are reports of problems or if there is an issue suggesting that one or more of the supplements are not safe. In

2004, the FDA removed supplements containing ephedra because of safety issues. In 2008, the FDA warned the public about approximately 69 weight-loss products, some of which claimed to be "natural" or "herbal," but that actually contained active, unapproved drug substances that were not food supplements. In 2009, multiple other products were withdrawn from the market.

Many feel that FDA regulation should be tighter. Although proposals have been made for stronger regulation, nothing has yet been put in place. Buyer beware.

In conclusion, over-the-counter weight-loss products that are dietary supplements are not regulated in the same manner as drugs, and safety and efficacy do not have to be proven. You should approach these products with caution. Usually few or no studies of these products exist, and long-term side effects are not known. If your child contemplates buying them, check the product and speak to your physician first. As these products are available in pharmacies or supermarkets without prescription, remember that your child can easily obtain them without your knowledge. Beware also of your child using one or more of these products without telling you.

It goes without saying (but will be said anyway) that street drugs, unlabeled pills or products, friends' drugs, and home-made concoctions should be totally avoided.

71. What is Alli? Is it okay to take?

Alli, which the FDA has reviewed and approved, is an over-the-counter, low-dose (60 mg) form of the drug (orlistat). It works by blocking the absorption of fat in the intestines, thus reducing the number of calories that get into the body. The nonabsorbed fat is eliminated in the stools. At a higher dose, orlistat is marketed by prescription only for weight loss. It was approved by the FDA in February 2007:

The Food and Drug Administration approved the drug product orlistat 60 mg capsule (trade name Alli) on February 7, 2007, for over-the-counter marketing as a weight loss aid. Alli is to be used only in conjunction with a weight loss program that includes a reduced calorie diet, a low fat diet, and an exercise program. It is approved for use in adults 18 years and older. A multivitamin should be taken every day when Alli is used as part of a weight loss program.

As the FDA noted, Alli should be used only in conjunction with a low-calorie, low-fat diet and an exercise program. It should not be used with the Atkins or any other high-fat/high-protein diet.

People who are not overweight, who have had an organ transplant, who are taking cyclosporine, or who have problems absorbing food should not take this drug. A multivitamin should be taken when using Alli. Side effects reported include gas with oily spotting, loose stools, and more frequent stools that may be hard to control. Cases of liver problems are being investigated by the FDA. If abdominal pain occurs, a doctor should be contacted immediately.

One capsule should be taken with each fat-containing meal. No more than three capsules should be taken per day. See the manufacturer's website (www.myalli.com) and the FDA approved drug labeling for further information as well as advice on diet and exercise.

No advice or information is given on how long the product should be taken. The manufacturer notes that

Alli may increase the weight loss of a diet and exercise by up to 50% compared with diet/exercise alone. Speak with your child's physician before using this drug.

72. Has the FDA approved any other over-the-counter products as safe and effective for weight loss or appetite suppression?

No.

73. What about prescription drugs? Which ones are approved? Should my child take one of them?

Three categories of FDA-approved drugs are available for weight loss in adults (not children). Each works in a different way. The oldest class is known as noradrenergic agents and includes drugs similar to amphetamines. The two newer classes are **serotonin** reuptake inhibitors and **lipase** inhibitors.

74. What are the noradrenergic agents?

Noradrenergic drugs work on the brain and have stimulating effects. The classic drug in this category is amphetamine. These drugs are "controlled drugs" (schedule II) and are habit forming and addictive. They are approved for only short-term use (a few weeks) and should not be used by people taking other stimulating drugs such as pseudoephedrine or other drugs such as furazolidone, guanadrel, guanethidine, or a monoamine oxidase inhibitor. Also, significant drug interactions are seen with antacids, carbonic anhydrase inhibitors, and other drugs.

Common side effects include fast heart rate, elevated blood pressure, palpitations, restlessness, insomnia, nervousness, euphoria, dry mouth, unpleasant taste,

---

Serotonin

A neurotransmitter found in the brain that seems to play a significant role in the control of appetite and certain moods such as depression and panic.

Lipase

An enzyme made by the pancreas that aids in the digestion of fats. Blocking this enzyme with a lipase inhibitor can cause fat malabsorption and weight loss.

Noradrenergic drugs

Drugs used in weight control that act on the brain and are stimulating. They are, in the United States, controlled drugs because they can be addicting. They can produce severe side effects.

blurred vision, heartburn, libido changes, confusion, diarrhea, dizziness, headache, abnormal heart rhythms, rash, abdominal pain, and fatigue. As noted, these drugs can cause physical and psychological dependence.

In the 1990s, the combination of phentermine (another noradrenergic drug) and fenfluramine or dexfenfluramine ("Fen-Phen") was popular for weight loss; however, cases of heart valve disease were seen. Fenfluramine and dexfenfluramine were removed from the market, and the use of this combination was stopped.

There is little or no experience with noradrenergic drugs in children for weight loss, and thus, these should generally not be used. If they are used, a physician with experience with the use of these drugs in children must follow the child closely.

75. What are serotonin-norepinephrine reuptake inhibitors? Aren't these used for depression and other psychiatric disease?

Serotonin-norepinephrine reuptake inhibitors are a newer class of drugs that work in the brain to increase the neurotransmitters (chemicals in the brain that transmit signals and information from one brain cell to another) serotonin and norepinephrine. The most common use of these drugs is in psychiatric diseases in adults and children. Serotonin-norepinephrine reuptake inhibitors are used for depression but are not approved by the FDA for use in children.

Sibutramine (Meridia) is the only FDA-approved drug in this category for weight loss; it is not approved for psychiatric diseases. The drug works by increasing the feeling of satiety, decreasing hunger, and stimulating resting energy use. It is approved for weight loss and the

Serotonin-norepinephrine reuptake inhibitors

Drugs that prevent brain cells from reabsorbing certain neurotransmitters, thus allowing these neurotransmitters to remain in the fluid-filled spaces around the nerves. These drugs have been used in the treatment of various psychiatric diseases, including depression.

Serotonin-norepinephrine reuptake inhibitors are used for depression but are not approved by the FDA for use in children.

maintenance of weight loss and should be used with a reduced-calorie diet. It is recommended for patients with a BMI of ≥ 30 or ≥ 27 if there are other risk factors such as diabetes, high lipids, and hypertension.

It should not be used by patients taking monoamine oxidase inhibitors, patients who have hypersensitivity to sibutramine or any of the inactive ingredients, patients who have a major eating disorder such as anorexia nervosa or bulimia nervosa, patients taking other centrally acting weight loss drugs, or patients with a history of certain heart diseases or strokes. It should not be used in pregnant women. Contraception is advised for women of childbearing age.

Side effects include high blood pressure, elevated pulse, seizures, bleeding, kidney or liver disorders, gallstones, decreased cognitive performance, and possibly pulmonary hypertension. Other side effects include dry mouth, constipation, and insomnia. Blood pressure and pulse should be checked periodically. Sibutramine may increase weight loss 5% to 10% in conjunction with diet and exercise. It has been used to keep weight off for up to 2 years. Long-term side effects, however, are not known.

Meridia is a controlled drug (schedule IV) and carries the risk of abuse and physical/psychological dependence. Physicians are instructed "to carefully evaluate patients for history of drug abuse and follow such patients closely, observing them for signs of misuse or abuse (e.g., drug development of tolerance, incrementation of doses, drug seeking behavior)."

The recommended starting dose in adults is 10 mg. It is administered once daily with or without food. If there is inadequate weight loss, the dose may be titrated after 4 weeks to a total of 15 mg once daily. The 5-mg dose should be reserved for patients who do not tolerate the 10-mg dose. A multivitamin should be taken daily.

Concerning use in children, the FDA-approved labeling states this: "The data are inadequate to recommend the use of sibutramine for the treatment of obesity in pediatric patients." In addition, other serotonin reuptake inhibitor drugs used to treat depression and other psychiatric problems "revealed a greater risk of . . . suicidal behavior or thinking during the first few months of treatment. . . . It is unknown if sibutramine increases the risk of suicidal behavior or thinking in pediatric patients." Clearly, this drug should be used with extreme caution in children and adolescents, obviously under the care of a physician with experience using this drug. Sibutramine cannot be used with a selective serotonin reuptake inhibitor (SSRI) such as citalopram, escitalopram, and others because of the risk of serotonin syndrome, a very serious side effect. Check with your child's physician.

76. What about lipase inhibitors? Are these the same as Alli?

Yes, Xenical (orlistat) is a lipase inhibitor and is the same medication as Alli (which is available over-the-counter at a lower dose). It is the only drug in this category that is available in the United States. The drug works by blocking the digestion (by the pancreas and stomach enzyme lipase) of dietary fat in the stomach and the small intestine. Unlike sibutramine and the noradrenergic inhibitor drugs, orlistat is minimally absorbed into the body from the intestines. Thus, unlike sibutramine and other drugs, it interacts with fewer other medications, and the side-effect picture is generally milder.

In clinical studies, adults using orlistat plus diet started losing weight within 2 weeks of starting and maintained it better at 1 year compared with control patients taking **placebo** plus diet. The studies suggest that orlistat plus diet allowed more patients to maintain a weight loss of more than 10% of body weight at 2 years compared with placebo plus diet.

Placebo

A "dummy" or inactive pill that is given as a comparative agent in a study of an active drug. Placebos should have no positive effect (efficacy) or negative effect (side effects), but they often do.

The most common side effects are oily spotting, flatus with discharge, fecal urgency, fatty/oily stool, oily evacuation, increased defecation, and fecal incontinence. FDA is examining possible liver problems seen with use of this drug. This medicate should not be used in patients with chronic malabsorption syndrome or cholestasis.

Unlike the other drugs, orlistat has been studied in children. In a study of over 300 adolescents 12 to 16 years old, on a well-balanced, reduced-calorie diet with a behavior-modification program and exercise counseling, about 65% completed the study. After 1 year of treatment, about 19% of the orlistat children compared with 12% of the placebo children had lost at least 5% of their body weight, and about 10% of the orlistat children lost more than 10% of their body weight compared with about 3% of the placebo children. The side effect profile was similar to that seen in adults.

You can read these results optimistically and say that the drug seems to help some of the children lose and maintain weight. On the other hand, only about 1 in 5 children lost more than 5% of their body weight at 1 year.

The approved, recommended dose is one 120-mg capsule three times a day, with each main meal containing fat. A multivitamin should be taken each day also. Obviously, work closely with your child's doctor if this drug is being used.

77. What is the difference between Alli and Xenical? Can I buy Alli and have my child use it at a higher dose without seeing the doctor?

Alli and Xenical contain the same drug (orlistat), with Alli containing 60 mg and Xenical 120 mg per pill. There are no head-to-head trials of the high and low dose. Although many drugs exhibit a "dose-response" effect (the higher the dose, the more effective it is but with more side effects), this has not been clearly studied with orlistat. In general, when taking a drug, the lowest effective dose is the best.

With an over-the-counter drug, the FDA has determined that your child does not need a "medical diagnosis," nor is your child necessarily followed by a physician or other medical practitioner. In contrast, a prescription drug requires that the patient speak with a physician (or in some jurisdictions a nurse practitioner or physician assistant), receive a prescription, and (again in some jurisdictions) have the opportunity to get advice from the pharmacist.

Thus, with Alli, you and/or your child can decide that his weight is too high and go buy the drug in a store or by mail or the Internet (from a legitimate pharmacy) without any medical advice. You and your child should read the label on the box or bottle and follow that advice. The dose should not be increased without speaking with your child's physician.

78. Are any other drugs available?

Other experimental drugs are in clinical trials but are not yet available. It is not clear whether they will be superior to the products currently available. Some have tried using other drugs already on the market to assist in weight loss. Drugs such as fluoxetine (Prozac), sertraline (Zoloft), and Bupropion (Wellbutrin, Zyban) have been tried. Some studies of these drugs have shown moderate, short-term weight loss on a diet–plus-medication program. Longer-term results are less clear with much weight regained after stopping the drug. These drugs must not be used at the same time as orlistat as a very serious side effect can occur.

Topiramate and Zonisamide, two FDA-approved drugs for seizures, have been used in weight loss, again with some modest success. Other drugs, including insulin-like compounds, have been studied, but nothing is currently on the horizon. At this point, all of these drugs are experimental and are not recommended for use in weight loss. If such an approach is desired, consider searching out a clinical trial for which your child might be eligible. Look at the U.S. government clinical trial registry at: www.clinicaltrials.gov.

There is one other drug that is not approved or available in the United States but is in other parts of the world including Europe. It is called rimonabant (Accomplia) and is a so-called cannabinoid receptor CB1 antagonist which works to suppress appetite. Clinical studies showing efficacy but side effects, particularly suicidal ideations, have prevented approval in the United States to date.

79. Has there been much controversy about these drugs?

Yes, there has been some controversy about these drugs. First, the results are only mild to moderate at best. As noted previously with orlistat (Xenical), at 1 year, fewer than 1 in 5 children had lost and maintained a weight of 5% or more. Side effects are rare, but an ongoing debate always exists about whether the benefits (weight loss) outweigh the risks (side effects). The evidence can be argued both ways with these drugs, although some feel that the risk of dependence with some of the drugs as well as the more severe side effect profile does not warrant their use except in extreme cases.

Various groups (including Public Citizen) have also made formal requests to the FDA to ban sibutramine totally from the market, as well as to not permit orlistat from moving (as it did) from prescription-only status to prescription (high dose) and over the counter (low dose).

On the other hand, others (including one drug manufacturer) have petitioned the FDA to declare that the claims that dietary supplements "promote, assist, or otherwise help in weight loss are disease claims." The effect of this would be to forbid such claims or possibly reclassify the supplements as drugs subject to tighter FDA regulation compared with food supplements (see Question 80). This would probably limit or decrease sales and usage. Part of this discussion hinges on claims that obesity is a disease and being overweight is not.

80. Are there any supplements such as fish oil, vitamins, or linoleic acid that will help my child lose weight?

No, none of these or other supplements has been shown to help in weight loss. Vitamins are necessary

Vitamins are necessary for good health, although again, none have been shown to help weight loss.

for good health, although again, none has been shown to help weight loss. Excess doses of certain vitamins can be harmful (particularly vitamins A, D, E, and K), whereas others are just excreted in the urine. The FDA has not approved these products for weight loss.

Actually, you should be very careful about any diet or food supplement marketed for diets, weight loss, appetite suppression, and so forth. As discussed in Question 70, the FDA regulates food and dietary supplements less tightly than it does conventional food and drugs. Most manufacturers of these products do not have to perform clinical trials to show that these products are safe and effective, nor do they have to submit any data to FDA. Similarly, the FDA does not check out most of these products before they come on the market. The FDA will react, however, if something appears to be a safety problem. For example, in 2008 and 2009, the FDA became aware of several potentially unsafe products (both imported and domestic). These were withdrawn from the market either by the company voluntarily or at the FDA's request.

See the FDA's website on dietary supplements: www.fda.gov/Food/DietarySupplements

81. What is the bottom line on drugs and dietary and weight-loss supplements?

Again, unfortunately, there is no magic bullet for losing weight. At best, the drugs and supplements may be a small help in a weight-loss and exercise program. The effects at best are small, and there is no clear evidence that they work after 1 or 2 years. The controlled drugs have clearly greater dependence/addiction risks and side-effect profiles and all must be used only under a physician's care. Enduring weight loss requires a lifestyle change with new and continued eating and exercise habits.

82. What about various surgeries? What are they? Do they work?

Yes, many techniques—from **liposuction** to stomach banding, to even more complex and invasive operations—exist. All surgery is obviously invasive to some degree, and all surgery carries risk—some greater than others. The techniques are also quite expensive and often not reimbursed by health insurance. In general, they are reserved for patients with massive obesity who have failed on conventional diets and drug therapy. They should not be done purely for cosmetic reasons. They are also considered in patients who have complications of obesity such as diabetes, hypertension, hyperlipidemia, joint disease, lung disease, or other serious disease.

Liposuction

A cosmetic surgical procedure to remove fatty tissue under the skin.

83. How about liposuction?

Liposuction (also called lipoplasty, fat modeling, liposculpture, lipectomy, lipo, or suction-assisted fat removal) is not a weight-loss technique. It is cosmetic surgery. It has no place in a weight-control program or lifestyle change. It is invasive and has significant side effects. Liposuction is generally done in people who are healthy and older than 18 years. Serious diseases (diabetes, heart problems, circulation problems, etc.) are contraindications to doing the procedure.

Multiple types of liposuction are available. Local, and sometimes general, anesthesia is needed. An antibiotic

Liposuction plays no role in your child's weight-loss program.

is given. The fat is removed and sutures placed. Side effects include bruising, swelling, pain, scarring, numbness, and (depending on where the procedure is done) limited mobility for a while. More serious complications can occur, including damage to surrounding tissue or skin, infection, clotting, bleeding, embolism, organ perforation, burns, and, rarely, death (data suggest a rate of 3 to 100 deaths per 100,000 procedures). See the FDA's website for further information (www.fda.gov/cdrh/liposuction/risks.html). Again, liposuction plays no role in your child's weight-loss program.

84. What other surgical techniques for weight loss or appetite control are available?

Many different types of surgery have been tried since the 1960s. They are usually reserved for patients with very marked obesity (e.g., a BMI over 40). Broadly speaking, two types of surgery are available (see Resources). The first is called restrictive, as it makes the stomach smaller and "restricts" the amount of food that can be eaten before the patient feels full. This limits meal size. The second type of surgery is more extensive and bypasses parts of the small intestine (where food is absorbed) to produce malabsorption of food. This bypass may also be combined with a restrictive procedure to prevent weight gain by both mechanisms.

Gastric banding

A surgical procedure designed to produce weight loss in which a band is put around the outside of the stomach to create a small pouch with limited capacity.

Gastric bypass

A surgical procedure designed to produce weight loss in which a surgeon disconnects part or all of the stomach so that food does not enter it.

Several of the more common procedures (from least invasive to most invasive) include:

- Adjustable **gastric banding**
- Vertical banded gastroplasty (gastric stapling)
- Roux-en-Y **gastric bypass** (RYGB)
- Biliopancreatic bypass

Multiple studies suggest that surgery can play a useful role in weight control in adults. There is very little information about the role of surgery in children. These are, however, largely "anecdotal reports" or uncontrolled trials. There are no adequate controlled trials of surgery versus medical therapy. One study in Sweden matched surgical patients with nonoperated patients (although this was not a true, classic, standard, prospective, randomized, controlled trial). Most of the patients were adult females with an average BMI of 41. The average weight loss for the surgical patients was about 44 pounds at 8 years compared with no change in the weight of the nonoperated patients. There was also a suggestion of improvements in high blood pressure, diabetes, blood lipid abnormalities, chest pain, shortness of breath, and quality of life, although not all improved at all time points.

Only a few studies have compared the actual surgical procedures with each other, and the results have suggested that bypass surgery produced greater weight loss; however, no procedure consistently proved to be superior.

Mortality rates generally have been looked at and most series suggest early mortality rates of 1% or less. One study found a 30-day mortality of 1.9%. As with many surgical procedures, there is a learning curve. Centers that did more procedures tended to report lower mortality and morbidity (side effect/complication) rates.

85. Can you describe the different surgical procedures possible? What is adjustable gastric banding?

Gastric banding is the least complex and the safest form of weight loss surgery, as there is no cutting of the stomach or intestines and recovery is rapid. A silicon band is

Gastric banding is the least complex and the safest form of weight loss surgery, as there is no cutting of the stomach or intestines and recovery is rapid.

wrapped around the upper part of the stomach to create a small pouch, which creates a very narrow channel leading into the lower part of the stomach. The band functions as a valve, allowing limited amounts of food and liquid to enter the lower parts of the stomach. After the band is placed, the stomach has, in effect, two parts and looks like an "hourglass" with a narrow waist and a small upper part. This upper stomach only holds an ounce or two before producing fullness and satiety. If more is eaten, nausea and vomiting will occur.

This procedure, unlike the more complex procedures described below, is called "restrictive," as it does not interfere with the normal digestion and absorption processes of the intestines. Rather, it restricts the amount of food that can be eaten and passed into the lower stomach and then the intestines.

Laparoscope

A tube passed through the skin into the abdomen allowing the doctor to view internal organs (with an attached camera) and perform surgical procedures without the need for a large incision.

This procedure is done through a **laparoscope** (a tube passed through the skin into the abdomen) using several small incisions. The band actually has a balloon valve filled with salt water that can be inflated (tightened) or deflated (loosened) to adjust the amount of food going into the lower part of the stomach. This is quite frequently done, as the surgeon can adjust or fine-tune the band to get the optimal weight loss with the fewest side effects. The FDA approved this procedure in 2001.

Weight loss can be from one-third to two-thirds of excess weight over about 2 years, and many keep the weight off for up to 5 years. Success rates can be as high as 70%, and this operation is practical and common for teens. As noted, adjustments of the band may be required from time to time. This is done in a couple of minutes in the surgeon's office.

Because the intestines are not cut and the normal anatomy and food flow through the intestines is not altered, there is no malabsorption or "dumping" (see Gastric Bypass in Question 87) or leaking. Surgery takes only an hour or two, and patients can usually resume their normal lives in a few days. As with the other procedures, the patient must develop a new lifestyle and way of eating—no more giant meals and no more eating quickly. Some foods must be chewed very well or even avoided, as they may not pass through the now-narrow stomach (e.g., dry bread and chicken). The procedure can be "defeated" if the patient eats and drinks very high-calorie foods (e.g., shakes and ice cream).

Side effects include movement, twisting, or slippage of the band or erosion of the band into the stomach. These may require a further laparoscopic procedure to correct. This is still surgery, and complications may occur. Death rates have been reported at 1 in 2,000.

This is one of the safest and easiest procedures for surgical weight loss in adolescents with severe, morbid obesity who have failed on diets and other nonsurgical programs.

86. What is gastric or stomach stapling?

This procedure is very similar to gastric banding. It uses a band and staples to create a small stomach pouch leading into the rest of the stomach. This is a more complex procedure than the banding procedure described in Question 85. In addition, the band is not adjustable. Although this stapling procedure is still done in some centers, it has largely been replaced by gastric banding. Problems can occur with the staples as well as with the band, which may become too narrow.

These usually require further surgery to correct the problem. Deaths have been reported.

87. What is the gastric bypass operation?

The gastric bypass is fairly extensive and alters the anatomy of the gastrointestinal tract. It is major abdominal surgery. The Roux-en-Y gastric bypass (RYGB) procedure involves first making the stomach smaller by stapling or by putting a band on to close the lower part of the stomach. The upper part of the stomach can then hold only a couple of ounces at most. Because the outlet from the bottom of the stomach into the **duodenum** (the uppermost part of the small intestine) is now closed, a new outlet must be created by bringing the **jejunum** (part of the small intestine) up to the new, small stomach pouch. This bypasses the rest of the stomach and the duodenum. The resulting shape is sort of a "Y," with the bottom of the stomach now being a dead end.

By doing this, the smaller stomach becomes full rapidly (creating satiety), so the patient eats smaller amounts of food. By bypassing the upper part of the small intestine, some of the ingested food and drink is not absorbed and passes out in the stool. This procedure can be done by a standard abdominal surgery technique with a large incision or, in some centers, by laparoscope involving a much smaller incision. Hospitalization for 2 to 7 days is required (the lower number for the laparoscopic procedure). In addition to the side effects and complications seen in any of these surgical procedures (e.g., infection, pain, and so forth), the **dumping syndrome** is seen with the bypass. The dumping syndrome is seen when the stomach contents (largely undigested) are rapidly moved ("dumped") into the small intestine. This causes nausea and

Duodenum

The uppermost part of the small intestine.

Jejunum

The part of the small intestine between the duodenum and the ileum.

Dumping syndrome

One of the side effects some patients experience after undergoing gastric bypass surgery. Undigested stomach contents are rapidly moved into the small intestine, causing nausea and vomiting, cramps, diarrhea, bloating, dizziness, rapid heart rate, anxiety, weakness, and fatigue.

vomiting, cramps, diarrhea, bloating, dizziness, rapid heart rate, anxiety, weakness, fatigue, and other symptoms. Some people get this soon after eating (within a few minutes) and others one to three hours later. Treatment includes changes in eating habits, medications, and, in severe cases, revision of the surgery. Mortality rates for the procedure are under 1.5%. Other longer-term side effects include iron and vitamin B_{12} deficiency (from poor absorption) requiring supplementation. Some patients develop narrowing at the junction between the stomach and the jejunum (**stomal stenosis**), loosening of the staples, or enlargement of the stomach pouch. Some patients develop ulcers and gallstones. If needed, the operation can be reversed, restoring the normal (more or less) anatomy.

Weight loss can occur quickly and can persist for one or more years, although weight may plateau and some may even be gained back.

Dr. Grant, bariatric surgeon, about Kim:

Kim is (or actually now was) a massively obese 16 year old with a BMI of over 42. She already has diabetes and, because she smokes, frequent bronchitis and pneumonia. She was hospitalized several times for these problems and once for depression. Because she has already developed significant health problems related to her weight and because she failed on multiple diets, she was placed in a residential school facility for 6 months. Because she also has a family history positive for cardiac disease, we felt that more aggressive measures were needed. I met with Kim alone and with her family several times and spoke with her pediatrician and nutritionist and psychiatrist, and we all agreed that surgery was the best option for her. She had the surgery last month, a gastric bypass, and recovered rapidly and completely. She's back at school, following

Stomal stenosis

A narrowing at the junction of two organs or "tubes." In the context of this book, producing some degree of obstruction to the passage of food.

her new lifestyle, losing weight, and is a different person from the Kim I saw before surgery. Her attitude has changed, and I think she now sees herself as becoming more "normal like the others at school," as she said to me. We are keeping a close eye on her because of the medical problems she had in the past. The next big step is to get her to stop smoking.

88. What is the biliopancreatic bypass (Scopinaro) procedure?

This too is major abdominal surgery. It was developed in Europe and is used more extensively there than in the United States. In this procedure, part of the stomach is removed, and a smaller stomach pouch remains. This pouch can be bigger than the one in the Roux-en-Y procedure. The pouch is connected much lower in the small intestine to the **ileum**. This bypasses the upper small intestine and means that less food is absorbed. In addition, the lower part of the stomach and duodenum (where bile and other fluids from the liver, gallbladder, and pancreas enter the intestines) is also attached to the lower part of the small intestine where these fluids enter the intestines. Several variations of this extensive procedure exist.

Ileum

The last part of the small intestine between the jejunum and the colon.

Because there is a bigger stomach pouch left than with the Roux-en-Y, more food can be eaten. All patients develop significant malabsorption (that is the purpose of the operation), and it is very effective for weight loss. Patients can lose up to two-thirds of their excess weight in 2 years (100 to 200 pounds). In some studies, excellent weight loss remains after many years.

The downside is that up to one-third of all patients have major complications requiring reoperation. About one-third of patients develop gallstones, and as a result, some surgeons will remove the gallbladder during surgery to lower this risk. Mortality can run 1% to 3% and, as with the other surgical procedures, is less common in more experienced centers.

Other complications can occur such as infection, wound breakdown, leaks, ulcers, and blood clots in the legs leading to pulmonary embolism. This can be seen in up to 10% of patients. A different lifestyle and diet must be followed. Because only about one-fourth of the ingested fat is absorbed, patients may have diarrhea with foul-smelling bowel movements and gas and bloating.

Clearly, this is extensive, complicated, and risky surgery and is reserved for only the most obese patients. Only part of the procedure is reversible. It is usually done with a large abdominal incision, although some centers are able to do it via laparoscope. This should be done only in a center where there is extensive experience with this surgery. This procedure is not common in children/teenagers. Most experts would advise one of the less extensive procedures such as banding first.

89. Are there any psychological or behavioral methods to help weight loss? Should my daughter see a behavioral therapist?

Yes, certain psychological methods can assist in weight loss and lifestyle change. The National Heart, Lung, and Blood Institute (NHLBI) has published its therapeutic guidelines for the treatment of obesity (see the Resources section for further information) in which they indicate that behavioral therapy plus diet can assist in short-term (less than 1 year) weight loss,

Behavioral therapy plus diet can assist in short-term (less than 1 year) weight loss, though the evidence for usefulness in longer-terms is not clear.

though the evidence for usefulness in longer-terms is not clear.

Behavioral therapy

A type of psychotherapy in which the patient is taught new techniques to modify certain negative behaviors by attempting to substitute new, learned positive behaviors in their place.

Behavioral therapy is a type of psychotherapy in which your child is taught new techniques to modify certain behaviors that produce and reinforce overeating and other bad habits and behaviors. It attempts to substitute new, learned behaviors for the bad ones that are producing weight gain and obesity. It aims to help your child understand thoughts and beliefs that are harmful or inappropriate. These thoughts and perceptions lead to negative reactions, emotions, and moods that are destructive. Behavioral therapy attempts to break this chain of negativity by showing how these thoughts are inaccurate and distorted and destructive. The attempt is then to replace them with useful, realistic, and helpful thoughts and then improved behaviors.

This therapy requires motivation on the part of your child (and you, the parents who are part of the support system), as the techniques learned during the therapy sessions must be used daily at home and integrated into her life and behavior. The techniques are safe and have no real side effects. For example, if there is weight loss, points can be given that will at some point be exchanged for a small reward such as going to a movie, quality time, etc.

To use these techniques, certain precepts must be accepted. If your daughter changes her diet and physical activity, she can lose weight. She can learn and use new ways to eat and exercise. She must change her environment in order for these new behaviors to be effective.

- Self-monitoring of both eating habits and physical activity—Keep a record of everything eaten and all physical activities.

- Stress management—Develop coping strategies to reduce stress.
- Stimulus control—Identify the stimuli and high-risk situations (e.g., going to candy stores) that cause bad eating.
- Problem solving—Develop ways to avoid the high-risk situations or stimuli that produce overeating.
- Contingency management—Use rewards for specific actions. For example, exercising four times a week for 6 months will earn a new MP-3 player. Sometimes rewards are simply verbal encouragement and support.
- Cognitive restructuring—Modify unrealistic goals, inaccurate beliefs, and self-defeating thoughts and feelings that undermine weight loss efforts. Replace excessive reactions ("I had fries and chocolate cake with lunch today. I blew it and I may as well give up my diet") with more reasonable ones ("I understand that what happened is not the end of the world and I can still continue to diet and lose weight").
- Social support—Get help from family, friends, support groups, and others. You may want to speak to your child's physician about such groups or look on the Internet for such therapists or support groups near you (see the Resources section).

From Bill, 15 years old:

What's the problem? I like to eat. I'm a little fat. Well, maybe more than a little, but I'm tall. My parents take me to a husky boys store or order nice clothes from some special place on the Internet. It doesn't matter though since I only wear jeans and t-shirts. I don't have to dress up for school or anything. The girls seem to like me, too, so I don't see what the big deal is. I eat what I want; I love fries and shakes and double cheeseburgers. I can eat a whole pizza for lunch. I don't even go to the school cafeteria for lunch.

They just serve veggies and fish and things. Nobody likes that stuff. The school nurse said that I might have health problems like my dad when I get older if I am still heavy. I don't smoke or use drugs, so I don't think I'll get sick. That doesn't worry me anyway, because I can lose the weight anytime I want. I just don't want to now.

90. Are there any psychological tricks to help with dieting?

Many people have published "tips" or "tricks" or "motivational aids" to help you lose weight. Here are some of them. It is not clear that they all work, but you may find some to be helpful. Keep in mind that some are actually contradictory, and some are "old wives tales" or "urban myths."

- Eat a lot of fruits and vegetables, as your diet allows.
- Don't skip meals, especially breakfast—even if you overdid it or "cheated" at an earlier meal that day or the day before. Just make them a little smaller than normal for a day or two. Skipping a meal may prevent activation of the satiety center several hours later and increase cravings.
- Don't mix different diets. Follow the rules set out in your diet.
- Mix different diets (a contradiction of the previous tip). Stay on one for a certain amount of time, and then switch to another one so that you don't get bored with the same foods all the time. (Actually, a good diet and new lifestyle should allow you to have lots of different foods, but pay attention to portion size and quantity.)
- Be realistic about goals and body image. Try to set reasonable goals and outcomes. Try to develop the understanding that you will never get the "perfect body."

- Also, be realistic about quick fixes and how much can be achieved in terms of weight loss. Understand that this is not a 100-yard dash but rather a marathon.
- Move around! Take the stairs two flights up and three flights down. Don't take the elevator. Walk the two blocks instead of taking the car.
- Snack smartly: vegetables, pretzels, yogurt, oranges, strawberries, apples, and pears—not potato chips and candy bars.
- Avoid refined sugar, bleached grains, and white flour.
- Don't forget that sugared drinks (cola) have calories.
- Limit caffeine drinks. Some people claim that they actually increase hunger.
- Drink lots of water.
- Avoid processed food.
- Eat food with lots of different tastes and textures.
- Imagine yourself after you've lost the weight and how you will look and how people will admire you. Use a motivational catch phrase like this: "Every day in every way I'm getting better and better."
- Eat meats that are 85% lean.
- Be positive.
- Eat alone sometimes, as it is claimed that people eat more when they eat with others.
- If others in your house are dieting, eat together to give each other moral support.
- Use a small plate for your food. It makes the portion look bigger.
- Eat foods that are moist and bulky and avoid dry foods.
- Don't even think of snacks for at least two hours after a meal.
- Get enough sleep.

- Try ethnic foods. They often taste quite differently from the normal diet and, if carefully chosen, may be very healthy and low in calories.
- If you feel hungry between meals, drink a glass of water. That may help the feeling pass.

91. Should I put my son into a program or group such as Weight Watchers or Jenny Craig or meal delivery programs?

Many programs are available to help with weight loss. They offer various levels of support (e.g., 24/7 phone support, group sessions, etc.), advice, and ongoing weight tracking, and some supply prepackaged meals. Most set reasonable goals and aim to get your BMI down over time to a healthy level (e.g., around 25 or less).

The Jenny Craig program has been around for many years and has centers around the United States. This program aims to change lifestyle and eating habits. In addition to support, they sell prepackaged food for three meals a day. These meals are based on the U.S. government Food Pyramid, with about 50% carbohydrate, 25% protein, and 25% fat. This is a low-calorie diet with portion control and exercise. There is a monthly cost as well as the cost of the prepackaged food and, if desired, various supplements.

Weight Watchers, a low-calorie and balanced diet, has also been around for many years and, like Jenny Craig, aims to change eating habits and lifestyle. Weight Watchers also has food that is sold in supermarkets. Rather than counting calories, Weight Watchers has developed a point system that combines calories, fat, and fiber content. You can have a certain number of points per day and can vary your foods. No food is forbidden, but portion size matters. Exercise is also encouraged as part of the healthy lifestyle. They, too, offer support and group meetings.

Nutrisystem is another program that offers prepackaged food based on low-calorie balanced (55% carbohydrate, 25% fat, and 20% protein) diets. It also encourages exercise.

These and others are national plans. You may find local plans, even those aimed particularly at children, advertised in your area that are similar to these. Also, compare prices, as they do vary. These plans tend to be reasonable and well done. They have stood the test of time and have many adherents. Remember that you will only hear the success stories. Go online to read some weight-loss forums to hear opinions of those who succeeded as well as those who failed.

To lose weight, you have to change your eating habits and lifestyle and do exercise. These programs can provide very useful assistance in doing this. They all tend to offer balanced, low-calorie menus that you either prepare yourself or purchase prepackaged. Some are delivered fresh daily (usually in big cities), and some are frozen food. With some, you can purchase food in supermarkets. As with any food that is prepared for you, however, the cost will be greater than preparing it yourself. Food can run up to $10 to $12 a day or more depending on whether you buy the "extras" and the supplements. There is also a charge for membership or meetings and support.

One criticism of the programs that supply prepackaged food is the "yo-yo effect" (see Question 92).

92. What is the yo-yo effect in dieting?

Yo-yo dieting is also called weight cycling. This refers to people who go on diets aimed at losing a lot of weight quickly. Although common in adults, it is seen in older children and adolescents who try to lose a lot of weight very quickly. This may involve "starvation" or very low-calorie diets (less than 800 to 1,000 calories per day) that produce rapid weight loss. When the diet is stopped and eating habits revert to prediet levels, the weight is gained right back. Part of this also involves the body's adaptation to the sudden drop in calories by slowing down metabolism. The body will use less energy per day, and weight loss will slow or even stop so that a plateau is reached and no changes occur in weight. To avoid this, the diet should not be drastic, and calorie intake per day should be calculated so that weight loss is limited to 1 to 2 pounds a week.

Some evidence shows that yo-yo dieting can be bad for one's health. Some people actually increase the amount of stored fat in the body after each weight gain part of the cycle. This occurs because during the weight-loss period both muscle and fat are lost. When the weight is regained, it tends to return more as fat than as muscle. Some soft evidence also shows that yo-yo dieting may have adverse effects on the immune system. Yo-yo dieting can also be quite distressing psychologically, as the patient may see this as a personal failure.

Yo-yoing is particularly likely if one's attitude is, "I'll do this diet until I lose my 20 pounds (or whatever number of pounds is chosen), and then I can stop dieting." If that occurs, then the weight will surely come back. The better attitude is, "I need to find a way of eating and a lifestyle that I can live with for the rest of my life—not for a fixed amount of time until the weight is lost."

You and your child must understand the unfortunate fact that life is not always fair. Some people can eat as much as they want and never gain weight. It seems, since you and your child are reading this book, that your child is *not* one of those people, which means you and your child will have to make some changes in order to arrive at and maintain a healthy weight.

93. My daughter said she'll do the diet for now but that she wants to return to her normal eating after she loses the weight. This doesn't sound wise. What should she do after the weight is lost?

You're right. With this attitude, the diet will not work, and she'll regain the weight after she stops dieting. She really does have to approach this as a change in habits and lifestyle and not a short-term diet. Going back to "normal" (i.e., the typical American teenager's eating style) really isn't normal or healthy. Your daughter needs to understand the concepts of portion control, balanced diets, and where calories come from (fat more than carbohydrates and proteins). She needs to understand that "cheating" only hurts her and that she "can't fool mother nature." Although she may undercount or ignore certain calories, her body won't.

Someone your daughter trusts and believes in needs to teach her this. This might be you, her doctor, the school nurse, a family member, or someone who has succeeded in losing weight and keeping it off. Only you and she can best determine who that should be.

94. My daughter goes out with her friends a lot, and they often end up at a fast-food place. What can she do? What should she eat when going out?

Depending on her diet, she will have to order food that fits her particular regimen. Clearly, at some places, it is harder to find healthy, reasonable dishes to order, but even at fast-food places, choices are available. She doesn't have to order the double cheeseburger with large fries and a shake. Many fast-food restaurants now have some lower calorie options on the menu as well as diet drinks without sugar. As noted in Question 49, a Big Mac, medium fries, and a shake can run over 1,500 calories. Getting a smaller burger, small fries (or no fries), and a diet soda will cut calories by as much as two-thirds.

95. Can my daughter cheat or slip? Can she go off the diet every now and then? What about vacations?

As noted in Question 94, everyone periodically has a meal out. Of course, everyone will go off the diet occasionally. Your daughter simply has to realize that calories are calories and that if she has too many today her weight loss will slow. As noted, "You can't cheat mother nature." If she wants to go off her diet for a meal, your daughter should just cut back (gently) at earlier or subsequent meals to make up for it. If she is a good exerciser, do a few more minutes on the treadmill or in the pool, but don't starve for a day. Just go back on the normal eating plan, and the extra calories will be "diluted" over the next few days.

Vacations can be very challenging indeed. At home, you have control of your food. You can shop, buy, prepare, and eat healthy foods. On vacation, in the car, at a hotel, or in a foreign country, you may not have much choice in what you eat. You may not see nutrition labels and have no idea what goes into the foods. Obviously, use common sense. If you do not eat fried foods much at home, do not eat them on the road. Try for fruits and salads and vegetables. Buy healthy snacks in advance for the car or plane so that you don't rely only on the (not always healthy) airplane or highway rest area foods. Where possible, bring food with you (e.g., a box of cereal or healthy snacks), and avoid buffet-style all-you-can-eat breakfasts and dinners.

96. My daughter has dieted before. She either doesn't lose the weight, or as soon as she stops the diet, she regains the weight. What can we do?

You and your daughter should try to understand why she failed and see whether there is some way to address the reason for failure when she tries again. You might want to consult with her doctor or a nutritionist. Did she try an unreasonable diet (e.g., starvation)? Did she understand that she is making a lifestyle change and not a 6-week food restriction plan after which she reverts to normal? Children often feel invincible and don't realize that choices and habits made now can affect them adversely for the rest of their lives. To comprehend this better, she may need additional help. Did she do the diet on her own, or did she have some structure? If on her own, perhaps she should try a program such as Weight Watchers (if you are willing to pay for this). Perhaps she could consult a dietitian or nutritionist and attend support groups. Low-calorie diets and a lifestyle change can be tough, particularly for adolescents and children who do not see or worry about future health issues that will likely arise (high blood pressure, heart disease, etc.). Explore diet programs at a nearby medical center, behavioral therapy support, prepackaged meals, and all of the other things mentioned in this book.

97. Are there comprehensive programs at medical centers that will help my son lose and maintain weight?

Yes, many medical centers and medical schools have such programs. Be sure to start with a program or specialist who is not a surgeon or does not immediately propose surgery. Unless there are very special circumstances (significant morbid obesity with a very high BMI), the first steps should always be nonsurgical.

Bariatrics

The branch of medicine and surgery that deals with the causes, prevention, management, and treatment of excess weight.

Some physicians specialize in weight loss medicine (**bariatric** medicine) and weight loss surgery (bariatric surgeons). Call a major medical center or medical school near you, and ask whether they have a weight-loss department or program, particularly for teens or adolescents. Also, ask your child's doctor.

You can find them on the Internet by searching such terms as:

- "Weight loss" "medical centers" "your county or town or city"
- Bariatric specialists "nonsurgeon"
- Dietitians, nutritionists, weight loss "your county or town or city"

As noted earlier, be very careful and check out anyone you find via the Internet or yellow pages. For physicians, look at their training, their hospital affiliations, and whether they are board certified in their field: in internal medicine and/or by the American Board of Physician Nutrition Specialists (ABPNS) and/or American Board of Nutrition (ABN). For nutritionists and dietitians, check for the following: registered dietitian (RD), certified nutrition support dietitian (CNSD), and/or specialist in pediatric nutrition (CSP).

98. What about weight-loss camps, residential programs, or boarding schools?

Many weight-loss camps (or spas) are available around the United States where adolescents and teens can go (usually for the summer) to develop healthy lifestyles. In addition to the usual summer camp activities, emphasis is on education about eating and healthy lifestyles. The goal is not just to lose some weight but also to understand how to eat and live moving forward so as not to regain the lost weight. Training is available in nutrition, exercise, eating (and sometimes cooking), goal setting, lifestyle choices, stress management, and other laudable topics. The goal is not massive weight loss during the summer, and these aren't "fat camps" or "boot camps." Usually the camps take children age 10 years and older, although some will take younger children.

Weight-loss schools are also beginning to appear. Most are boarding schools at the high school level, although some may be day schools where the students live at home as normal. These schools do the normal academic teaching but also add further information on stress management, weight loss, and nutrition and provide support and counseling for dieting and lifestyle change. Of course, the cafeteria food is carefully monitored. Check with your child's school guidance counselor or nurse or administrator or check on the Internet. As always, be sure to check thoroughly any

Many weight-loss camps (or spas) are available around the United States where adolescents and teens can go (usually for the summer) to develop healthy lifestyles.

Treatment

schools or camps found via the Internet or yellow pages or advertising.

99. What role should the school play in our son's weight-loss program?

The public and educators are finally beginning to join in the fight against childhood obesity. Offering better meals in the cafeteria, limiting access to vending machines, providing healthy snacks, and other measures are slowly being put into effect. There is more teaching of nutrition and good lifestyle behavior. Required physical activity is still spotty but is recognized as a critical part of a healthy lifestyle.

In 2007, the U.S. Institute of Medicine, a nonprofit institution chartered by the U.S. National Academy of Sciences, published a report with excellent recommendations for nutrition in the schools. Food in schools comes from three sources: food the children bring in, food served in the lunchroom or cafeteria, and "competitive" foods sold in vending machines or elsewhere. Obviously, food brought into the school cannot easily be controlled short of policing lunch and breakfast. Food served in school is covered under current federal guidelines and recommendations for school nutrition.

These recommendations cover "competitive" food sold and are available in schools. The goal is to increase the eating of fruits, vegetables, and grains and to decrease salt, sugar, and saturated fat foods.

Discuss these guidelines, and look at the school menus (which are often distributed to students and parents) to see whether they are indeed healthy. Have a look at the vending machines and food sold competitively. See whether nutrition and healthy lifestyle instruction is included in any of the coursework and how much physical education is provided. If you feel there are inadequacies, speak with the school administrators, principal, and others on the board of education to lobby for help in the fight against childhood obesity. You will likely find very willing allies.

100. So what is the bottom line for my child?

You've come this far—congratulations! Hopefully you have learned a lot about your child's weight problem. Let's sum up.

If your child is at the right weight (BMI less than the 75th percentile) and living and eating a healthy lifestyle, congratulations! If your child is at risk, that is, a BMI in the 75th to 84th percentile, then be sure that you and your child are aware of good nutrition habits and the appropriate weight and lifestyle to maintain. Speak with your child's physician. You may want to have your child visit a nutritionist once or twice a year to be sure that he or she is following a healthy diet and lifestyle. You may also want to consider having your child see a behavior therapist and exercise physiologist or trainer to assist in moving to or maintaining a good lifestyle.

If your child is in the 85th to 95th percentile, then definitely see the nutritionist and behavior therapist and trainer a couple of times a year to be sure that your child understands and follows a good diet and lifestyle. Definitely speak with your child's physician.

Finally, if he or she is above the 95th percentile, you and your child need to take strong action. See the doctor and/or nutritionist, and be sure that your child is on a healthy, balanced reducing diet with exercise and behavioral training. It is critical to do this so that he or

If your child is overweight or obese, he or she really needs to slim down slowly over time and adopt good living habits that will last a lifetime and will serve you well.

she does not become an overweight or obese adult with all of the health problems that come with that.

If your child is overweight or obese, he or she really needs to slim down slowly over time and adopt good living habits that will last a lifetime and will serve you well.

Good luck!

Organizations

American Dietetic Association Get Nutrition Fact Sheets
American Dietetic Association
Consumer Education Team
216 West Jackson Boulevard
Chicago, IL 60606
http://www.eatright.org

American Obesity Association
1250 24th Street, NW, Suite 300
Washington, DC 20037
Phone: (800) 98-OBESE
http://www.obesity.org

American Society of Bariatric Physicians (ASBP)
5600 S. Quebec, Suite 109-A
Englewood, CO 80111
Phone: (303) 779-4833, (303) 770-2526
Fax: (303) 779-4834
http://www.asbp.org

The Council on Size and Weight Discrimination—An advocacy group
P.O. Box 305
Mt. Marion, NY 12456
http://www.cswd.org

U.S. Food and Drug Administration (FDA)
10903 New Hampshire Avenue
Silver Spring, MD 20993
Phone: (888) INFO-FDA, (888) 463-6332
http://www.fda.gov

Shape Up America!—A nonprofit organization
http://www.shapeup.org/index.php

Many more resources are available on the Internet. Search online for topics of interest, but as always, check carefully any site or organization that you link to or contact.

Support Groups

NYU: http://thinforlife.med.nyu.edu/surgicalweightloss/supportgroups/
Stony Brook (SUNY): www.stonybrookmedicalcenter.org/body.cfm?id=1753
Kansas City: www.childrensmercy.org/Content/view.aspx?id=5856

Carefully check out any group you might want to use at:
http:// www.bsciresourcecenter.com

Websites

American Academy of Pediatrics policy statement on childhood obesity:
http://pediatrics.aappublications.org/cgi/reprint/112/2/424

American Academy of Pediatrics report for healthcare practitioners on the concept of staged diagnosis, assessment, and treatment of obesity in children:
http://pediatrics.aappublications.org/cgi/reprint/120/Supplement_4/S164

American College of Physicians pharmacologic and surgical management of obesity in primary care:
http://www.annals.org/cgi/reprint/142/7/525.pdf

BMI Calculators:
http://pediatrics.about.com/cs/usefultools/l/bl_bmi_calc.htm
http://www.healthline.com/sw/clc-childrens-bmi-calculator
http://www.nhlbisupport.com/bmi

Centers for Disease Control on childhood obesity:
http://www.cdc.gov/HealthyYouth/obesity

Calories per activity calculators (by body weight, age, and gender):
http://www.health.drgily.com/basal-metabolic-rate-calculator.php
http://www.fit4lifeclub.com/tools/calories-burned-per-day.html

Dallas Dietetic Association calorie counter:
http://www.dallasdietitian.com/resources/calcalc.asp?result=2896

Endocrine Society Clinical Practice Guideline:
http://jcem.endojournals.org/cgi/content/abstract/93/12/4576

Food and Drug Administration learning program on weight loss and nutrition:
http://www.fda.gov/loseweight

Food and Drug Administration information on contaminated weight-loss
products:
www.fda.gov/ForConsumers/ConsumerUpdates/ucm136187.htm

Food diaries:
http://www.familydoctor.org/online/famdocen/home/healthy/food/general-
nutrition/299.html
http://www.weightloss.about.com/cs/ourtoptips/l/blfooddiary.htm

Harvard School of Public Health nutrition guidelines:
http://www.hsph.harvard.edu/nutritionsource/what-should-you-eat/
carbohydrates-full-story/index.html

Ideal body weight calculator:
http://pediatrics.about.com/cs/growthcharts2/l/bl_ibw_calc.htm

Low-carbohydrate diet plans:
http://www.lowcarb.ca/atkins-diet-and-low-carbplans

The Mayo Clinic on childhood obesity:
http://www.mayoclinic.com/health/childhood-obesity/DS00698

National Institutes of Health guidebook outlining various strategies that are
useful in behavioral therapy:
http://www.nhlbi.nih.gov/guidelines/obesity/e_txtbk/txgd/4323.htm

***Pediatrics* report on prevention and treatment of childhood obesity:**
http://pediatrics.aappublications.org/cgi/reprint/120/Supplement_4/S164

U.S. Department of Agriculture "My Pyramid" website with details on the Food
Pyramid with dietary guidelines as well as sites for parents, preschoolers, and kids:
http://www.mypyramid.gov

**U.S. Institute of Medicine Committee on Progress in Preventing Childhood
Obesity Report:**
http://iom.edu/CMS/3788/25044.aspx

U.S. Institute of Medicine report on school nutrition standards:
http://www.iom.edu/Object.File/Master/42/505/Food%20in%20Schools.pdf

Weight-loss surgeries:
New York University Medical Center:
http://www.thinforlife.med.nyu.edu/obesitysurgery
The Department of Health and Human Services:
http://www.win.niddk.nih.gov/publications/gastric.htm
The American Medical Association:
http://www.jama.ama-assn.org/cgi/reprint/294/15/1986.pdf
The Nemours Foundation (aimed at teens contemplating surgery):
http://www.kidshealth.org/teen/diseases_conditions/obesity/bariatric.html
American Society for Bariatric Surgery:
http://www.asbs.org
British Obesity Surgery Patient Association:
http://www.bospa.org/Information.aspx?Page=2

Research Studies

Childhood obesity, prevalence and prevention. *Nutrition Journal* http://www.nutritionj.com/content/4/1/24
Early life risk factors for obesity in childhood: cohort study. *British Medical Journal.* http://www.bmj.com/cgi/content/full/330/7504/1357
Environmental influences on childhood obesity: ethnic and cultural influences in context. *Physiology & Behavior.* http://www.find-health-articles.com/rec_pub_18158165-environmentalinfluences-childhood-obesity-ethnic-cultural-influences.htm
Low-dose leptin reverses skeletal muscle, autonomic, and neuroendocrine adaptations to maintenance of reduced weight. *Journal of Clinical Investigation.* http://www.jci.org/articles/view/25977
Parents' awareness of overweight in themselves and their children. *British Medical Journal.* http://www.bmj.com/cgi/content/full/330/7481/23
40-year follow-up of overweight children. *Department of Pediatrics, University Hospital, Linköping, Sweden.* http://www.ncbi.nlm.nih.gov/pubmed/2570196?dopt=Abstract

Dietary Guidelines for Americans

U.S. Department of Agriculture

U.S. Department of Health and Human Services and U.S. Department of Agriculture. *Dietary Guidelines for Americans, 2005*, 6th ed. Washington, DC: U.S. Government Printing Office, January 2005. www.health.gov/DietaryGuidelines/dga2005/document/default.htm

Executive Summary

The *Dietary Guidelines for Americans (Dietary Guidelines)* provides science-based advice to promote health and to reduce risk for major chronic diseases through diet and physical activity. Major causes of morbidity and mortality in the United States are related to a poor diet and a sedentary lifestyle. Some specific diseases linked to poor diet and physical inactivity include cardiovascular disease, type 2 diabetes, hypertension, osteoporosis, and certain cancers. Furthermore, poor diet and physical inactivity, resulting in an energy imbalance (more calories consumed than expended), are the most important factors contributing to the increase in overweight and obesity in this country. Combined with physical activity, following a diet that does not provide excess calories according to the recommendations in this document should enhance the health of most individuals.

An important component of each 5-year revision of the *Dietary Guidelines* is the analysis of new scientific information by the Dietary Guidelines Advisory Committee (DGAC) appointed by the Secretaries of the U.S. Department of Health and Human Services (HHS) and the U.S. Department of Agriculture (USDA). This analysis, published in the DGAC Report (www.health.gov/dietaryguidelines/dga2005/report/), is the primary resource for development of the report on the Guidelines by the Departments. The *Dietary Guidelines* and the report of the DGAC differ in scope and purpose compared to reports for previous versions of the *Guidelines*. The 2005 DGAC report is a detailed scientific analysis. The scientific report was used to develop the *Dietary Guidelines* jointly between the two departments and forms the basis of recommendations that will be used by USDA and HHS for program and policy development. Thus it is a publication oriented toward policymakers, nutrition educators, nutritionists, and healthcare providers rather than to the general public, as with previous versions of the *Dietary Guidelines*, and contains more technical information.

The intent of the *Dietary Guidelines* is to summarize and synthesize knowledge regarding individual nutrients and food components into recommendations for a pattern of eating that can be adopted by the public. In this publication, key recommendations are grouped under nine interrelated focus areas. The recommendations are based on the preponderance of scientific evidence for lowering risk of chronic disease and promoting health. It is important to remember that these are integrated messages that should be implemented as a whole. Taken together, they encourage most Americans to eat fewer calories, be more active, and make wiser food choices.

A basic premise of the *Dietary Guidelines* is that nutrient needs should be met primarily through consuming foods. Foods provide an array of nutrients and other compounds that may have beneficial effects on health. In certain cases, fortified foods and dietary supplements may be useful sources of one or more nutrients that otherwise might be consumed in less than recommended amounts. However, dietary supplements, while recommended in some cases, cannot replace a healthful diet.

Two examples of eating patterns that exemplify the *Dietary Guidelines* are the USDA Food Guide (www.usda.gov/cnpp/pyramid.html) and the DASH (Dietary Approaches to Stop Hypertension) Eating Plan.[1] Both of these eating patterns are designed to integrate dietary recommendations into a healthy way to eat for most individuals. These eating patterns are not weight loss diets, but rather illustrative examples of how to eat in accordance with the *Dietary Guidelines*. Both eating patterns are constructed across a range of calorie levels to meet the needs of various age and gender groups. For the USDA Food Guide, nutrient content estimates for each food group and subgroup are based on population-weighted food intakes. Nutrient content estimates for the DASH Eating Plan are based on selected foods chosen for a sample 7-day menu. While originally developed to study the effects of an eating pattern on the prevention and treatment of hypertension, DASH is one example of a balanced eating plan consistent with the 2005 *Dietary Guidelines*.

Throughout most of this publication, examples use a 2,000-calorie level as a reference for consistency with the Nutrition Facts Panel. Although this level is used as a reference, recommended calorie intake will differ for individuals based on age, gender, and activity level. At each calorie level, individuals who eat nutrient-dense foods may be able to meet their recommended nutrient intake without consuming their full calorie allotment. The remaining calories—*the discretionary calorie allowance*—allow individuals flexibility to consume some foods and beverages that may contain added fats, added sugars, and alcohol.

The recommendations in the *Dietary Guidelines* are for Americans over 2 years of age. It is important to incorporate the food preferences of different racial/ethnic groups, vegetarians, and other groups when planning diets and developing educational programs and materials. The USDA Food Guide and the DASH Eating Plan are flexible enough to accommodate a range of food preferences and cuisines.

The *Dietary Guidelines* is intended primarily for use by policymakers, healthcare providers, nutritionists, and nutrition educators. The information in the *Dietary Guidelines* is useful for the development of educational materials and aids policymakers in designing and implementing nutrition-related programs, including federal food, nutrition education, and information programs. In addition, this publication has the potential to provide authoritative statements as provided for in the Food and Drug Administration Modernization Act (FDAMA). Because the *Dietary Guidelines* contains discussions where the science is emerging, only statements included in the Executive Summary and the sections titled "Key Recommendations," which reflect the preponderance of scientific evidence, can be used for identification of authoritative statements. The recommendations are interrelated and mutually dependent; thus the statements in this document should be used together in the context of planning an overall healthful diet. However, even following just some of the recommendations can have health benefits.

The following is a listing of the *Dietary Guidelines* by chapter.

ADEQUATE NUTRIENTS WITHIN CALORIE NEEDS

Key Recommendations

- Consume a variety of nutrient-dense foods and beverages within and among the basic food groups while choosing foods that limit the intake of saturated and *trans* fats, cholesterol, added sugars, salt, and alcohol.
- Meet recommended intakes within energy needs by adopting a balanced eating pattern, such as the USDA Food Guide or the DASH Eating Plan.

Key Recommendations for Specific Population Groups

- *People over age 50.* Consume vitamin B_{12} in its crystalline form (i.e., fortified foods or supplements).
- *Women of childbearing age who may become pregnant.* Eat foods high in heme-iron and/or consume iron-rich plant foods or iron-fortified foods with an enhancer of iron absorption, such as vitamin C-rich foods.
- *Women of childbearing age who may become pregnant and those in the first trimester of pregnancy.* Consume adequate synthetic folic acid daily (from fortified foods or supplements) in addition to food forms of folate from a varied diet.
- *Older adults, people with dark skin, and people exposed to insufficient ultraviolet band radiation (i.e., sunlight).* Consume extra vitamin D from vitamin D-fortified foods and/or supplements.

WEIGHT MANAGEMENT

Key Recommendations

- To maintain body weight in a healthy range, balance calories from foods and beverages with calories expended.
- To prevent gradual weight gain over time, make small decreases in food and beverage calories and increase physical activity.

Key Recommendations for Specific Population Groups

- *Those who need to lose weight.* Aim for a slow, steady weight loss by decreasing calorie intake while maintaining an adequate nutrient intake and increasing physical activity.
- *Overweight children.* Reduce the rate of body weight gain while allowing growth and development. Consult a healthcare provider before placing a child on a weight-reduction diet.
- *Pregnant women.* Ensure appropriate weight gain as specified by a healthcare provider.
- *Breast-feeding women.* Moderate weight reduction is safe and does not compromise weight gain of the nursing infant.
- *Overweight adults and overweight children with chronic diseases and/or on medication.* Consult a healthcare provider about weight loss strategies prior to starting a weight-reduction program to ensure appropriate management of other health conditions.

PHYSICAL ACTIVITY

Key Recommendations

- Engage in regular physical activity and reduce sedentary activities to promote health, psychological well-being, and a healthy body weight.
  - To reduce the risk of chronic disease in adulthood: Engage in at least 30 minutes of moderate-intensity physical activity, above usual activity, at work or home on most days of the week.
  - For most people, greater health benefits can be obtained by engaging in physical activity of more vigorous intensity or longer duration.

- ○ To help manage body weight and prevent gradual, unhealthy body weight gain in adulthood: Engage in approximately 60 minutes of moderate- to vigorous-intensity activity on most days of the week while not exceeding caloric intake requirements.
- ○ To sustain weight loss in adulthood: Participate in at least 60 to 90 minutes of daily moderate-intensity physical activity while not exceeding caloric intake requirements. Some people may need to consult with a healthcare provider before participating in this level of activity.
- Achieve physical fitness by including cardiovascular conditioning, stretching exercises for flexibility, and resistance exercises or calisthenics for muscle strength and endurance.

Key Recommendations for Specific Population Groups

- *Children and adolescents.* Engage in at least 60 minutes of physical activity on most, preferably all, days of the week.
- *Pregnant women.* In the absence of medical or obstetric complications, incorporate 30 minutes or more of moderate-intensity physical activity on most, if not all, days of the week. Avoid activities with a high risk of falling or abdominal trauma.
- *Breast-feeding women.* Be aware that neither acute nor regular exercise adversely affects the mother's ability to successfully breastfeed.
- *Older adults.* Participate in regular physical activity to reduce functional declines associated with aging and to achieve the other benefits of physical activity identified for all adults.

FOOD GROUPS TO ENCOURAGE

Key Recommendations

- Consume a sufficient amount of fruits and vegetables while staying within energy needs. Two cups of fruit and 2 1/2 cups of vegetables per day are recommended for a reference 2,000-calorie intake, with higher or lower amounts depending on the calorie level.

- Choose a variety of fruits and vegetables each day. In particular, select from all five vegetable subgroups (dark green, orange, legumes, starchy vegetables, and other vegetables) several times a week.
- Consume 3 or more ounce-equivalents of whole-grain products per day, with the rest of the recommended grains coming from enriched or whole-grain products. In general, at least half the grains should come from whole grains.
- Consume 3 cups per day of fat-free or low-fat milk or equivalent milk products.

Key Recommendations for Specific Population Groups

- *Children and adolescents.* Consume whole-grain products often; at least half the grains should be whole grains. Children 2 to 8 years of age should consume 2 cups per day of fat-free or low-fat milk or equivalent milk products. Children 9 years of age and older should consume 3 cups per day of fat-free or low-fat milk or equivalent milk products.

FATS

Key Recommendations

- Consume less than 10% of calories from saturated fatty acids and less than 300 mg/day of cholesterol, and keep *trans* fatty acid consumption as low as possible.
- Keep total fat intake between 20% and 35% of calories, with most fats coming from sources of polyunsaturated and monoun-saturated fatty acids, such as fish, nuts, and vegetable oils.
- When selecting and preparing meat, poultry, dry beans, and milk or milk products, make choices that are lean, low fat, or fat free.
- Limit intake of fats and oils high in saturated and/or *trans* fatty acids, and choose products low in such fats and oils.

Key Recommendations for Specific Population Groups

- *Children and adolescents.* Keep total fat intake between 30% and 35% of calories for children 2 to 3 years of age and between 25%

and 35% of calories for children and adolescents 4 to 18 years of age, with most fats coming from sources of polyunsaturated and monounsaturated fatty acids, such as fish, nuts, and vegetable oils.

CARBOHYDRATES

Key Recommendations
- Choose fiber-rich fruits, vegetables, and whole grains often.
- Choose and prepare foods and beverages with little added sugars or caloric sweeteners, such as amounts suggested by the USDA Food Guide and the DASH Eating Plan.
- Reduce the incidence of dental caries by practicing good oral hygiene and consuming sugar- and starch-containing foods and beverages less frequently.

SODIUM AND POTASSIUM

Key Recommendations
- Consume less than 2,300 mg (approximately 1 tsp of salt) of sodium per day.
- Choose and prepare foods with little salt. At the same time, consume potassium-rich foods, such as fruits and vegetables.

Key Recommendations for Specific Population Groups
- *Individuals with hypertension, African Americans, and middle-aged and older adults.* Aim to consume no more than 1,500 mg of sodium per day, and meet the potassium recommendation (4,700 mg/day) with food.

ALCOHOLIC BEVERAGES

Key Recommendations
- Those who choose to drink alcoholic beverages should do so sensibly and in moderation—defined as the consumption of up to one drink per day for women and up to two drinks per day for men.

- Alcoholic beverages should not be consumed by some individuals, including those who cannot restrict their alcohol intake, women of childbearing age who may become pregnant, pregnant and lactating women, children and adolescents, individuals taking medications that can interact with alcohol, and those with specific medical conditions.
- Alcoholic beverages should be avoided by individuals engaging in activities that require attention, skill, or coordination, such as driving or operating machinery.

FOOD SAFETY

Key Recommendations
- To avoid microbial food-borne illness:
  - Clean hands, food contact surfaces, and fruits and vegetables. Meat and poultry should not be washed or rinsed.
  - Separate raw, cooked, and ready-to-eat foods while shopping, preparing, or storing foods.
  - Cook foods to a safe temperature to kill microorganisms.
  - Chill (refrigerate) perishable food promptly and defrost foods properly.
  - Avoid raw (unpasteurized) milk or any products made from unpasteurized milk, raw or partially cooked eggs or foods containing raw eggs, raw or undercooked meat and poultry, unpasteurized juices, and raw sprouts.

Key Recommendations for Specific Population Groups
- *Infants and young children, pregnant women, older adults, and those who are immunocompromised.* Do not eat or drink raw (unpasteurized) milk or any products made from unpasteurized milk, raw or partially cooked eggs or foods containing raw eggs, raw or undercooked meat and poultry, raw or undercooked fish or shellfish, unpasteurized juices, and raw sprouts.
- *Pregnant women, older adults, and those who are immunocompromised:* Only eat certain deli meats and frankfurters that have been reheated to steaming hot.

NIH Publication No. 03-4082, Facts about the DASH Eating Plan, United States Department of Health and Human Services, National Institutes of Health, National Heart, Lung, and Blood Institute. Karanja NM, et al. *Journal of the American Dietetic Association (JADA)* 8:S19–S27, 1999. www.nhlbi.nih.gov/health/public/heart/hbp/dash/.

DIETARY GUIDELINES FOR AMERICANS: APPENDIX A: EATING PATTERNS

www.health.gov/dietaryguidelines/dga2005/document/html/appendixA.htm

Appendix A-1: The DASH Eating Plan at 1,600-, 2,000-, 2,600-, and 3,100-Calorie Levels[a]

The DASH eating plan is based on 1,600, 2,000, 2,600, and 3,100 calories. The number of daily servings in a food group vary depending on caloric needs (see Table 3 to determine caloric needs). This chart can aid in planning menus and food selection in restaurants and grocery stores (Table A-1).

Appendix A-2: USDA Food Guide

The suggested amounts of food to consume from the basic food groups, subgroups, and oils to meet recommended nutrient intakes at 12 different calorie levels. Nutrient and energy contributions from each group are calculated according to the nutrient-dense forms of foods in each group (e.g., lean meats and fat-free milk). Table A-2 also shows the discretionary calorie allowance that can be accommodated within each calorie level, in addition to the suggested amounts of nutrient-dense forms of foods in each group.

Notes for Appendix A-2

[1] Food items included in each group and subgroup:

- Fruits: All fresh, frozen, canned, and dried fruits and fruit juices, for example, oranges and orange juice, apples and apple juice, bananas, grapes, melons, berries, raisins. In developing the food patterns, only

Food Groups	1,600 Calories	2,000 Calories	2,600 Calories	3,100 Calories	Serving Sizes	Examples and Notes	Significance of Each Food Group to the DASH Eating Plan
Grains[b]	6 servings	6–8 servings	10–11 servings	12–13 servings	1 slice bread, 1-ounce dry cereal,[c] 0.5-cup cooked rice, pasta, or cereal	Whole wheat bread, English muffin, pita, bread, bagel, cereals, grits, oatmeal, crackers, unsalted pretzels, and popcorn	Major sources of energy and fiber
Vegetables	3–4 servings	4–5 servings	5–6 servings	6 servings	1 cup raw leafy vegetable, 0.5-cup cutup raw or cooked vegetable, 0.5-cup vegetable juice	Tomatoes, potatoes, carrots, green peas, squash, broccoli, turnip greens, collards, kale, spinach, artichokes, green beans, lima beans, sweet potatoes	Rich sources of potassium, magnesium, and fiber
Fruits	4 servings	4–5 servings	5–6 servings	6 servings	1 medium fruit; 0.25-cup dried fruit; 0.5-cup fresh, frozen, or canned fruit; 0.5-cup vegetable juice	Apricots, bananas, dates, grapes, oranges, orange juice, grapefruit, grapefruit juice, mangoes, melons, peaches, pineapples, prunes, raisins, strawberries, tangerines	Important sources of potassium, magnesium, and fiber
Fat-free or low-fat milk and milk products	2–3 servings	2–3 servings	3 servings	3–4 servings	1-cup milk, 1-cup yogurt, 1.5-oz cheese	Fat-free or low-fat milk or buttermilk, fat-free or low-fat regular or frozen yogurt, fat-free, low-fat, or reduced fat cheese	Major sources of calcium and protein

					Serving sizes	Examples and notes	Significance
Lean meats, poultry and fish	3–4 servings	6 or less servings	6 servings	6–9 servings	1-oz cooked meats, poultry, or fish, 1 egg[d]	Select only lean; trim away visible fats; broil, roast, or boil instead of frying; remove skin from poultry	Rich sources of protein and magnesium
Nuts, seeds, and legumes	3–4 servings/ week	4–5 servings/ week	1 serving	1 serving	1/3 cup or 1.5-oz nuts; 2-tablespoons peanut butter; 2-tablespoons or 0.5-oz seeds; 0.5-cup cooked dry beans or peas	Almonds, filberts, mixed nuts, peanuts, walnuts, sunflower seeds, kidney beans, lentils	Rich sources of energy, magnesium, potassium, protein, and fiber
Fat and oils[e]	2 servings	2–3 servings	3 servings	4 servings	1-teaspoon soft margarine, 1-tablespoon mayonnaise, 2-tablespoons salad dressing, 1-teaspoon vegetable oil	Soft margarine, low-fat mayonnaise, light salad dressing, vegetable oil (such as olive, corn, canola, or safflower)	The DASH study had 27 percent of calories as fat (low in saturated fat), including fat in or added to foods
Sweets	0 servings	5 or less servings/ week	2 or less servings	2 or less servings	1-tablespoon sugar, 1-tablespoon jelly or jam, 0.5-cup sorbet and ices, 1-cup lemonade	Maple syrup, sugar, jelly, jam, fruit-flavored gelatin, hard candy, fruit punch, sorbet, and ices	Sweets should be low in fat

[a] www.nhlbi.nih.gov; Karanja NM et al. *JADA* 8:S19–S27, 1999.

[b] Whole grains are recommended for most grain servings to meet fiber recommendations.

[c] Equals 0.5 to 1.25 cups, depending on cereal type. Check the product's Nutrition Facts Label.

[d] Because eggs are high in cholesterol, limit egg yolk intake to no more than four per week; two egg whites have the same protein content as 1 ounce of meat.

[e] Fat content changes serving counts for fats and oils: for example, 1 tablespoon of regular salad dressing equals one serving; 1 tablespoon of a low-fat dressing equals 0.5 serving; 1 tablespoon of a fat-free dressing equals 0 servings.

This table is updated to reflect 2006 DASH Eating Plan.

Table A-2 USDA Food Guide

Daily Amount of Food From Each Group (vegetable subgroup amounts are per week)

Calorie Level	1,000	1,200	1,400	1,600	1,800	2,000
Food Group[1]	Food group amounts shown in cup (c) or ounce-equivalents (oz-eq), with number of servings (srv) in parentheses when it differs from the other units. See note for quantity equivalents for foods in each group[2]. Oils are shown in grams (g).					
Fruits	1 c (2 srv)	1 c (2 srv)	1.5 c (3 srv)	1.5 c (3 srv)	1.5 c (3 srv)	2 c (4 srv)
Vegetables[3]	1 c (2 srv)	1.5 c (3 srv)	1.5 c (3 srv)	2 c (4 srv)	2.5 c (5 srv)	2.5 c (5 srv)
Dark green vegetable	1 c/wk	1.5 c/wk	1.5 c/wk	2 c/wk	3 c/wk	3 c/wk
Orange vegetable	.5 c/wk	1 c/wk	1 c/wk	1.5 c/wk	2 c/wk	2 c/wk
Legumes	.5 c/wk	1 c/wk	1 c/wk	2.5 c/wk	3 c/wk	3 c/wk
Starchy vegetable	1.5 c/wk	2.5 c/wk	2.5 c/wk	2.5 c/wk	3 c/wk	3 c/wk
Other vegetable	4 c/wk	4.5 c/wk	4.5 c/wk	5.5 c/wk	6.5 c/wk	6.5 c/wk
Grains[4]	3 oz-eq	4 oz-eq	5 oz-eq	5 oz-eq	6 oz-eq	6 oz-eq
Whole grains	1.5	2	2.5	3	3	3
Other grains	1.5	2	2.5	2.5	3	3
Lean meat and beans	2 oz-eq	3 oz-eq	4 oz-eq	5 oz-eq	5 oz-eq	5.5 oz-eq
Milk	2 c	2 c	2 c	3 c	3 c	3 c
Oils[5]	15 g	17 g	17 g	22 g	24 g	27 g

Discretionary calorie allowance[6]	165	171	171	132	195	267
Calorie Level	2,200	2,400	2,600	2,800	3,000	3,200
Fruits	2 c (4 srv)	2 c (4 srv)	2 c (4 srv)	2.5 c (5 srv)	2.5 c (5 srv)	2.5 c (5 srv)
Vegetables[3]	3 c (6 srv)	3 c (6 srv)	3.5 c (7 srv)	3.5 c (7 srv)	4 c (8 srv)	4 c (8 srv)
Dark green vegetable	3 c/wk	3 c/wk	3 c/wk	3 c/wk	3 c/wk	3 c/wk
Orange vegetable	2 c/wk	2 c/wk	2.5 c/wk	2.5 c/wk	2.5 c/wk	2.5 c/wk
Legumes	3 c/wk	3 c/wk	3.5 c/wk	3.5 c/wk	3.5 c/wk	3.5 c/wk
Starchy vegetable	6 c/wk	6 c/wk	7 c/wk	7 c/wk	9 c/wk	9 c/wk
Other vegetable	7 c/wk	7 c/wk	8.5 c/wk	8.5 c/wk	10 c/wk	10 c/wk
Grains[4]	7 oz-eq	8 oz-eq	9 oz-eq	10 oz-eq	10 oz-eq	10 oz-eq
Whole grains	3.5	4	4.5	5	5	5
Other grains	3.5	4	4.5	5	5	5
Lean meat and beans	6 oz-eq	6.5 oz-eq	6.5 oz-eq	7 oz-eq	7 oz-eq	7 oz-eq
Milk	3 c	3 c	3 c	3 c	3 c	3 c
Oils[5]	29 g	31 g	34 g	36 g	44 g	51 g
Discretionary calorie allowance[6]	290	362	410	426	512	648

fruits and juices with no added sugars or fats were used. See Note 6 on discretionary calories if products with added sugars or fats are consumed.

- Vegetables: In developing the food patterns, only vegetables with no added fats or sugars were used. See Note 6 on discretionary calories if products with added fats or sugars are consumed.
  - Dark green vegetables: All fresh, frozen, and canned dark green vegetables, cooked or raw: for example, broccoli; spinach; romaine; collard, turnip, and mustard greens.
  - Orange vegetables: All fresh, frozen, and canned orange and deep yellow vegetables, cooked or raw: for example, carrots, sweet potatoes, winter squash, and pumpkin.
  - Legumes: All cooked dry beans and peas and soybean products: pinto beans, kidney beans, lentils, chickpeas, and tofu (dry beans and peas) (see comment under meat and beans group about counting legumes in the vegetable or the meat and beans group).
  - Starchy vegetables: All fresh, frozen, and canned starchy vegetables: for example, white potatoes, corn, and green peas.
- Grains: In developing the food patterns, only grains in low-fat and low-sugar forms were used. See Note 6 on discretionary calories if products that are higher in fat and/or added sugars are consumed.
  - Whole grains: All whole-grain products and whole grains used as ingredients: for example, whole-wheat and rye breads, whole-grain cereals and crackers, oatmeal, and brown rice.
  - Other grains: All refined grain products and refined grains used as ingredients: for example, white breads, enriched grain cereals and crackers, enriched pasta, and white rice.

See Note 6 on discretionary calories if higher fat products are consumed. Dry beans and peas and soybean products are considered part of this group as well as the vegetable group, but should be counted in one group only.

- Milk, yogurt, and cheese (milk): All milks, yogurts, frozen yogurts, dairy desserts, cheeses (except cream cheese), including lactose-free and lactose-reduced products. Most choices should be fat free or low fat. In developing the food patterns, only fat-free milk was used. See Note 6 on discretionary calories if low-fat, reduced-fat, or whole milk or milk products that contain added sugars are consumed. Calcium-fortified soy beverages are an option for those who want a nondairy calcium source.

[2]Quantity equivalents for each food group:

- Grains: The following each count as 1-ounce equivalent (1 serving) of grains: cup cooked rice, pasta, or cooked cereal; 1 ounce dry pasta or rice; 1 slice bread; 1 small muffin; 1 cup ready-to-eat cereal flakes.
- Fruits and vegetables The following each count as 1 cup (servings) of fruits or vegetables: 1 cup cut-up raw or cooked fruit or vegetable, 1 cup fruit or vegetable juice, 2 cups leafy salad greens.
- Meat and beans—The following each count as 1 ounce-equivalent: 1 ounce lean meat, poultry, or fish; 1 egg; $1/4$ cup cooked dry beans or tofu; 1 Tbsp peanut butter; $1/2$ ounce nuts or seeds.
- Milk—The following each count as 1 cup (1 serving) of milk: 1 cup milk or yogurt, $1^1/_2$ ounces natural cheese such as cheddar cheese, or 2 ounces processed cheese. Discretionary calories must be counted for all choices, except fat-free milk.

[3]Explanation of vegetable subgroup amounts: Vegetable subgroup amounts are shown in this table as weekly amounts because it would be difficult for consumers to select foods from each subgroup daily. A daily amount that is one seventh of the weekly amount listed is used in calculations of nutrient and energy levels in each pattern.

[4]Explanation of grain subgroup amounts: The whole-grain subgroup amounts shown in this table represent at least three 1-ounce servings and one half of the total amount as whole grains for all calorie levels of 1,600 and above. This is the minimum suggested amount of whole grains to consume as part of the food patterns. More whole grains up to all of the grains recommended may be selected, with offsetting decreases in the amounts of other (enriched) grains. In patterns designed for younger children (1,000, 1,200, and 1,400 calories), one half of the total amount of grains is shown as whole grains.

[5]Explanation of oils: *trans* fat, shown in this table represent the amounts that are added to foods during processing, cooking, or at the table. Oils and soft margarines include vegetable oils and soft vegetable oil table spreads that have no *trans* fats. The amounts of oils listed in this table are not considered to be part of discretionary calories because they are a major source of the vitamin E and polyunsaturated fatty acids, including the

essential fatty acids, in the food pattern. In contrast, solid fats are listed separately in the discretionary calorie table (Appendix A-3) because, compared with oils, they are higher in saturated fatty acids and lower in vitamin E and polyunsaturated and monounsaturated fatty acids, including essential fatty acids. The amounts of each type of fat in the food intake pattern were based on 60% oils and/or soft margarines with no *trans* fats and 40% solid fat. The amounts in typical American diets are about 42% oils or soft margarines and about 58% solid fats.

[6]Explanation of discretionary calorie allowance: The discretionary calorie allowance is the remaining amount of calories in each food pattern after selecting the specified number of nutrient-dense forms of foods in each food group. The number of discretionary calories assumes that food items in each food group are selected in nutrient-dense forms (that is, forms that are fat-free or low fat and that contain no added sugars). Solid fat and sugar calories always need to be counted as discretionary calories, as in the following examples:

- The fat in low-fat, reduced-fat, or whole-milk or milk products or cheese and the sugar and fat in chocolate milk, ice cream, pudding, etc.
- The fat in higher fat meats (e.g., ground beef with more than 5% fat by weight, poultry with skin, higher fat luncheon meats, sausages)
- The sugars added to fruits and fruit juices with added sugars or fruits canned in syrup
- The added fat and/or sugars in vegetables prepared with added fat or sugars
- The added fats and/or sugars in grain products containing higher levels of fats and/or sugars (e.g., sweetened cereals, higher fat crackers, pies and other pastries, cakes, cookies)

Total discretionary calories should be limited to the amounts shown in the table at each calorie level. The number of discretionary calories is lower in the 1,600-calorie pattern than in the 1,000-, 1,200-, and 1,400-calorie patterns. These lower calorie patterns are designed to meet the nutrient needs of children 2 to 8 years old. The nutrient goals for the 1,600-calorie pattern are set to meet the needs of adult women, which are higher and require that more calories be used in selections from the basic food groups. Additional information about discretionary calories, including an example

Table A-3 Discretionary Calorie Allowance in the USDA Food Guide

Discretionary Calories That Remain at Each Calorie Level												
Food Guide calorie level	1,000	1,200	1,400	1,600	1,800	2,000	2,200	2,400	2,600	2,800	3,000	3,200
Discretionary calories[1]	165	171	171	132	195	267	290	362	410	426	512	648
Example of division of discretionary calories: solid fats are shown in grams (g) and added sugars in grams (g) and teaspoons (tsp).												
Solid fats[2]	11 g	14 g	14 g	11 g	15 g	18 g	19 g	22 g	24 g	24 g	29 g	34 g
Added sugars[3]	20 g (5 tsp)	16 g (4 tsp)	16 g (4 tsp)	12 g (3 tsp)	20 g (5 tsp)	32 g (8 tsp)	36 g (9 tsp)	48 g (12 tsp)	56 g (14 tsp)	60 g (15 tsp)	72g (18 tsp)	96 g (24 tsp)

of the division of these calories between solid fats and added sugars, is provided in Appendix A-3.

Appendix A-3. Discretionary Calorie Allowance in the USDA Food Guide

The discretionary calorie allowance is the remaining amount of calories in each calorie level after nutrient-dense forms of foods in each food group are selected. Table A-3 shows the number of discretionary calories remaining in each calorie level if nutrient-dense foods are selected. Those trying to lose weight may choose not to use discretionary calories. For those wanting to maintain their weight, discretionary calories may be used to increase the amount of food selected from each food group; to consume foods that are not in the lowest fat form (such as 2% milk or medium-fat meat) or that contain added sugars; to add oil, fat, or sugars to foods; or to consume alcohol. Table A-3 shows an example of how these calories may be divided between solid fats and added sugars.

[1]Discretionary calories: In developing the Food Guide, food items in nutrient-dense forms (that is, forms that are fat-free or low-fat and that contain no added sugars) were used. The number of discretionary calories assumes that food items in each food group are selected in nutrient-dense forms. Solid fat and sugar calories always need to be counted as discretionary calories, as in the following examples:

- The fat in low-fat, reduced-fat, or whole milk or milk products or cheese and the sugar and fat in chocolate milk, ice cream, pudding, etc.
- The fat in higher fat meats (e.g., ground beef with more than 5% fat by weight, poultry with skin, higher fat luncheon meats, sausages)
- The sugars added to fruits and fruit juices with added sugars or fruits canned in syrup
- The added fat and/or sugars in vegetables prepared with added fat or sugars

- The added fats and/or sugars in grain products containing higher levels of fats and/or sugars (e.g., sweetened cereals, higher fat crackers, pies and other pastries, cakes, cookies)

Total discretionary calories should be limited to the amounts shown in the table at each calorie level. The number of discretionary calories is lower in the 1,600-calorie pattern than in the 1,000-, 1,200-, and 1,400-calorie patterns. These lower calorie patterns are designed to meet the nutrient needs of children 2 to 8 years old. The nutrient goals for the 1,600-calorie pattern are set to meet the needs of adult women, which are higher and require that more calories be used in selections from the basic food groups. The calories assigned to discretionary calories may be used to increase intake from the basic food groups; to select foods from these groups that are higher in fat or with added sugars; to add oils, solid fats, or sugars to foods or beverages; or to consume alcohol. See Note 2 on limits for solid fats.

[2]Solid fats: Amounts of solid fats listed in Table A-3 represent about 7% to 8% of calories from saturated fat. Foods in each food group are represented in their lowest fat forms, such as fat-free milk and skinless chicken. Solid fats shown in this table represent the amounts of fats that may be added in cooking or at the table, and fats consumed when higher fat items are selected from the food groups (e.g., whole milk instead of fat-free milk, chicken with skin, or cookies instead of bread), without exceeding the recommended limits on saturated fat intake. Solid fats include meat and poultry fats eaten either as part of the meat or poultry product or separately; milk fat such as that in whole milk, cheese, and butter; shortenings used in baked products; and hard margarines. Solid fats and oils are separated because their fatty acid compositions differ. Solid fats are higher in saturated fatty acids, and commonly consumed oils and soft margarines with no *trans* fats are higher in vitamin E and polyunsaturated and monounsaturated fatty acids, including essential fatty acids. Oils listed in Appendix A-2 are not considered part of the discretionary calorie allowance because they

are a major source of the essential fatty acids and vitamin E in the food pattern.

The gram weights for solid fats are the amounts of these products that can be included in the pattern and are not identical to the amount of lipids in these items because some products (margarines, butter) contain water or other ingredients, in addition to lipids.

[3]Added sugars: Added sugars are the sugars and syrups added to foods and beverages in processing or preparation, not the naturally occuring sugars in fruits or milk. The amounts of added sugars suggested in the example are *not* specific recommendations for amounts of added sugars to consume, but rather represent the amounts that can be included at each calorie level without over-consuming calories. The suggested amounts of added sugars may be helpful as part of the Food Guide to allow for some sweetened foods or beverages, without exceeding energy needs. This use of added sugars as a calorie balance requires two assumptions: (1) that selections are made from all food groups in accordance with the suggested amounts and (2) that additional fats are used in the amounts shown, which together with the fats in the core food groups, represent about 27% to 30% of calories from fat.

Height, Weight, and BMI Percentiles for Children

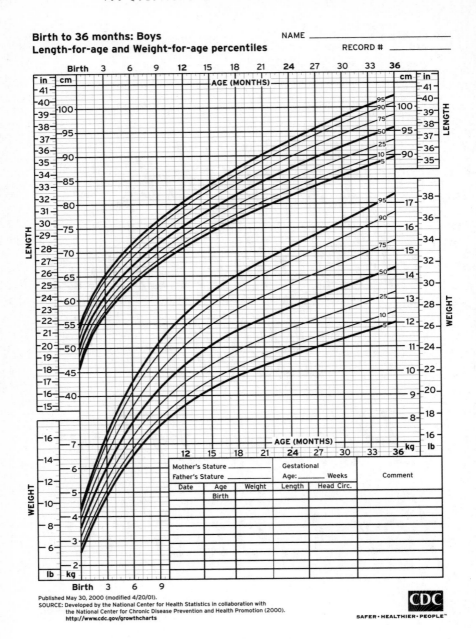

Birth to 36 months: Boys
Length-for-age and Weight-for-age percentiles

NAME _____

RECORD # _____

Published May 30, 2000 (modified 4/20/01).
SOURCE: Developed by the National Center for Health Statistics in collaboration with
the National Center for Chronic Disease Prevention and Health Promotion (2000).
http://www.cdc.gov/growthcharts

CDC
SAFER · HEALTHIER · PEOPLE™

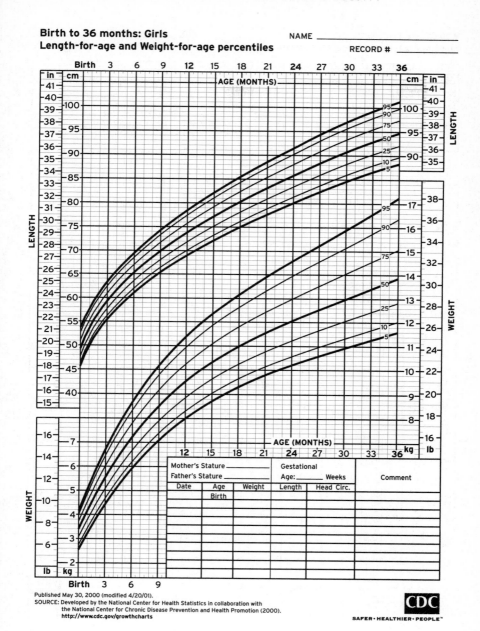

Birth to 36 months: Girls
Length-for-age and Weight-for-age percentiles

NAME _____

RECORD # _____

Published May 30, 2000 (modified 4/20/01).
SOURCE: Developed by the National Center for Health Statistics in collaboration with
the National Center for Chronic Disease Prevention and Health Promotion (2000).
http://www.cdc.gov/growthcharts

CDC
SAFER·HEALTHIER·PEOPLE™

Appendix B

2 to 20 years: Boys
Body mass index-for-age percentiles

NAME _____

RECORD # _____

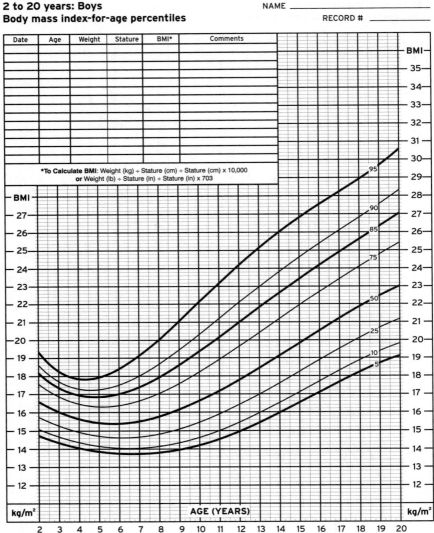

*To Calculate BMI: Weight (kg) ÷ Stature (cm) ÷ Stature (cm) x 10,000
or Weight (lb) ÷ Stature (in) ÷ Stature (in) x 703

AGE (YEARS)

Published May 30, 2000 (modified 10/16/00).
SOURCE: Developed by the National Center for Health Statistics in collaboration with
the National Center for Chronic Disease Prevention and Health Promotion (2000).
http://www.cdc.gov/growthcharts

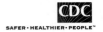

SAFER·HEALTHIER·PEOPLE™

2 to 20 years: Girls
Body mass index-for-age percentiles

NAME _____

RECORD # _____

Published May 30, 2000 (modified 10/16/00).
SOURCE: Developed by the National Center for Health Statistics in collaboration with
the National Center for Chronic Disease Prevention and Health Promotion (2000).
http://www.cdc.gov/growthcharts

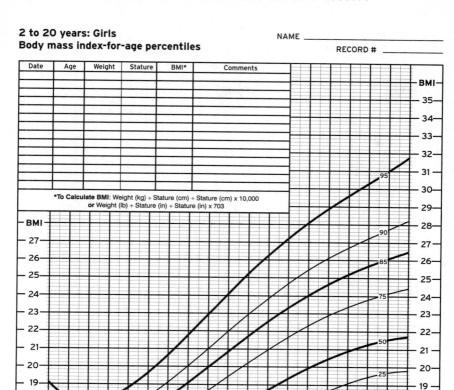

SAFER · HEALTHIER · PEOPLE™

Appendix B

165

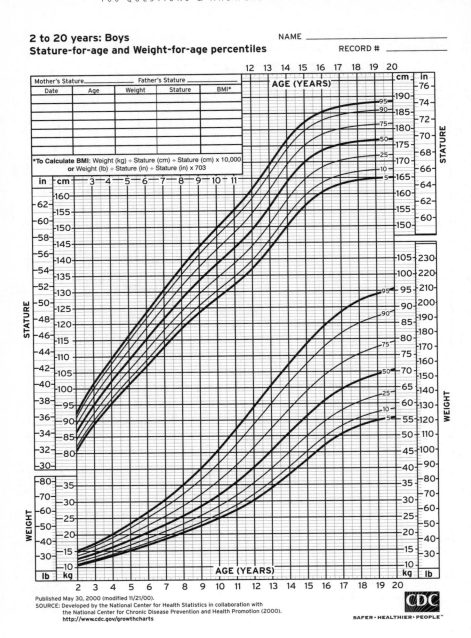

2 to 20 years: Boys
Stature-for-age and Weight-for-age percentiles

NAME _____

RECORD # _____

Published May 30, 2000 (modified 11/21/00).
SOURCE: Developed by the National Center for Health Statistics in collaboration with
the National Center for Chronic Disease Prevention and Health Promotion (2000).
http://www.cdc.gov/growthcharts

SAFER · HEALTHIER · PEOPLE™

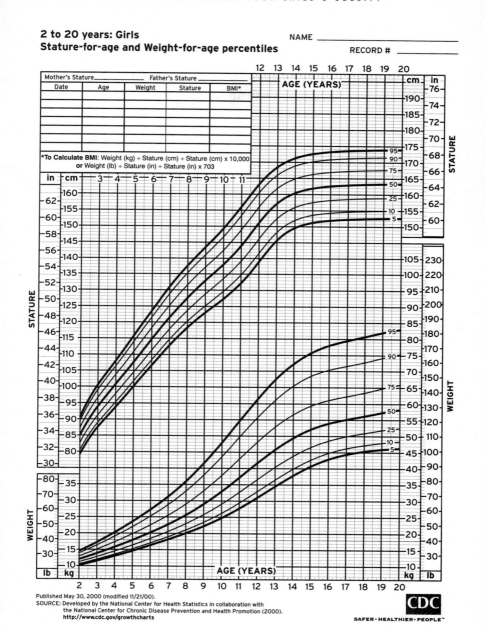

2 to 20 years: Girls
Stature-for-age and Weight-for-age percentiles

NAME _____

RECORD # _____

Appendix B

Published May 30, 2000 (modified 11/21/00).
SOURCE: Developed by the National Center for Health Statistics in collaboration with
the National Center for Chronic Disease Prevention and Health Promotion (2000).
http://www.cdc.gov/growthcharts

CDC
SAFER · HEALTHIER · PEOPLE™

Glossary

Adenoviruses: A group of viruses that affect mainly children. They can produce gastrointestinal and respiratory infections as well as urinary and eye infections.

Adiponectin: A hormone produced by fat cells that plays a role in the uptake, production, and storage of glucose, as well as fat metabolism.

Adipose: Fat cells. There are two types: white and brown.

Anorexia nervosa: A potentially very serious disease that can be fatal. It is characterized by excess weight loss and emaciation even though the patient may perceive herself to be "fat." This disease is more common in females than males, and can lead to some patients starving to death.

Asthma: A common disease of the breathing tubes (airways) in which reversible narrowing occurs producing difficulty in breathing. It can range from mild to severe and can be fatal.

Atherosclerosis: A common disease in which plaque (a combination of cholesterol, calcium and other compounds) builds up inside the inner walls of arteries. It can produce obstruction of these arteries leading to heart attacks, strokes and other significant medical problems.

Attention deficit/hyperactivity disorder: A behavioral disease usually seen in children characterized by impulsiveness, over-activity (hyperactivity) and poor attention/concentration.

Bardet-Biedl syndrome: A rare familial, recessively transmitted genetic disorder. The clinical characteristics of this syndrome include impaired vision or even blindness, extra fingers, a diminished or missing sense of smell, disease of the heart muscle, abnormalities with the reproductive and urinary systems, mental and developmental abnormalities, and obesity.

Bariatrics: The branch of medicine and surgery that deals with the causes, prevention, management, and treatment of excess weight.

Basal metabolic rate: The minimum energy needed or used by the body at complete rest to stay alive (keeping the heart pumping, breathing, blood circulating, and so forth).

Behavioral therapy: A type of psychotherapy in which the patient is taught new techniques to modify certain negative behaviors by attempting to substitute new, learned positive behaviors in their place.

Binge eating: A disorder in which the patient eats large and excessive amounts of food at periodic or occasional intervals. As these patients usually do not vomit after a binge, they may gain large amounts of weight. Binge eating may be seen in other disorders.

Bioelectrical impedance: A highly accurate way to measure a person's body mass. A small electric current, which flows at different rates through fat and fat-free tissues, is sent through the body. When factors such as height, weight, and gender are analyzed with the results, a measure of a person's body fat can be obtained.

Blount's disease: An abnormal bowing of the legs that occurs in children. While the exact cause is unknown, obesity is one risk factor for this condition.

Body mass index (BMI): A number calculated from height and weight that is used to determine whether a person is in the "normal" weight, underweight, overweight, or obese range.

Bulimia nervosa: A disease of binge eating followed by self-induced purges (vomiting, laxative use, enemas) to get rid of the food just eaten. This can lead to serious heart, kidney, and other diseases as well as depression. Fatal cases have been reported.

Calories: Units of energy. Although there is a technical definition (the amount of heat needed to raise one kg of water one degree Celsius at sea level), in the context of this book, it refers to the amount of energy in a food or the amount of energy that a person used.

Carbohydrate: One of the three main sources of energy for the body. These are compounds made up of carbon, hydrogen, and oxygen and include sugars, starches, celluloses, and gums. There are several types based on size and shape: monosaccharides, disaccharides, trisaccharides, polysaccharides, and heterosaccharides. They are a key source of energy for the body. Each gram of carbohydrate has four calories.

Celiac disease: A disease of the small intestine in which gluten containing foods are not tolerated producing diarrhea and other gastrointestinal symptoms. It is also called "nontropical sprue" or "gluten intolerance."

Cholecystokinin: A hormone secreted in the intestines that aids in fat digestion by causing the gall bladder to contract and release bile into the gut as well as causing the pancreas to release digestive hormones. It is also found in the brain as a neurotransmitter where it has entirely different functions.

Cholelithiasis: A disease in which there are stones in the gall bladder and/or common bile duct.

Cholesterol: A fat (lipid) that is an essential part of the membranes of cells. It is made by the body as well as ingested with food. It is a steroid and is necessary for life, but an excess can produce atherosclerosis leading to vascular and other diseases including heart attacks and strokes.

Chromosome: Thread-like structures containing genes found in the DNA of a cell. There are 23 pairs of chromosomes in human cells.

Compulsive eating disorder: A condition in which patients cannot control how much or how often they eat. They often feel anxious or panicked while eating, then guilt or depression after. It has also been called an addiction to food.

Coronary artery (heart) disease: A disease of the arteries of the heart in which the deposition of plaque (cholesterol, calcium, and other compounds) progressively blocks the flow of blood to the heart, which can lead to chest pain (angina pectoris) and myocardial infarction (heart attack).

Diabetes mellitus: A complex disease of small blood vessels and glucose metabolism. It is manifested by elevated levels of sugar (glucose) in the blood. Long-term adverse consequences include kidney failure, cataracts, poor circulation leading to heart attacks, strokes, leg ulcers, and other serious problems.

Dumping syndrome: One of the side effects some patients experience after undergoing gastric bypass surgery. Undigested stomach contents are rapidly moved into the small intestine, causing nausea and vomiting, cramps, diarrhea, bloating, dizziness, rapid heart rate, anxiety, weakness, and fatigue.

Duodenum: The uppermost part of the small intestine.

Endocrine disrupters: Compounds or other external products taken into the body that can interfere with normal body function and may alter a person's weight-control mechanisms. Sometimes casually called "obesogens."

Endothelium: A thin layer of cells that lines the inside of blood and lymph vessels as well as other body cavities.

Fat: See also lipids. One gram of fat contains and produces nine calories of energy. As an adjective and colloquially, it refers to being overweight or obese.

Flat feet: A medical condition in which the arch of the foot collapses, causing the entire sole of the foot to be in contact with the ground. There is some data that people who are overweight or obese are at greater risk of developing flat feet.

Gastric banding: A surgical procedure designed to produce weight loss in which a band is put around the outside of the stomach to create a small pouch with limited capacity.

Gastric bypass: A surgical procedure designed to produce weight loss in which a surgeon disconnects part or all of the stomach so that food does not enter it.

Genes: Units of DNA within a chromosome that can produce a protein having a particular function or producing a change in the body.

Genetic disorder: A disease or abnormality in the body due to a problem in the DNA (gene, chromosome) of a person or organism that is inherited.

Ghrelin: A hormone produced in the stomach, pancreas, and brain that seems to stimulate appetite.

Glucagon: A hormone that the body uses to regulate blood sugar, helping raise it when it is low.

Glucose: A simple sugar (carbohydrate) found in the body and easily measured in the blood.

Glycemic index: A number score given to carbohydrates as a function of how high and how quickly they raise blood sugar and insulin. Scores below 55 are low, meaning that they raise blood sugar slowly; scores above 70 cause a rapid rise in blood sugar.

Glycemic load: A calculation based on the glycemic index multiplied by the number of grams of carbohydrates, all of which is then multiplied by 100. This is an extension of the glycemic index in that it accounts for the amount of carbohydrates eaten and is useful in meal planning.

Glycogen: A complex sugar (carbohydrate) that the body makes from many glucose molecules chained together. It is used to store energy for later use.

Hepatic steatosis: A condition where excess fat builds up in liver cells. It can be caused by obesity, diabetes, or excessive use of alcohol. Also called fatty liver.

High-density lipoprotein (HDL) cholesterol: "Good cholesterol." The lipoproteins help carry the cholesterol to the liver for excretion from the body.

Hormones: Chemicals produced and secreted by glands, which then act at a distant site in the body.

Hyperlipidemia: An excess of one or more lipids in the blood that can lead to heart disease, strokes, and other medical problems.

Hypertension: An elevation of the pressures in the heart and arteries, which can lead to severe disease including heart attacks and strokes. Also called high blood pressure.

Hypogonadism: Poorly developed or incomplete sexual organs.

Hypothalamus: A part of the brain below the thalamus that controls such body functions as sleep, temperature, and appetite.

Hypothyroidism: Decreased thyroid function. This can produce weight gain, low energy levels, anemia, constipation, dizziness, hair loss, irregular menses, and other problems.

Ileum: The last part of the small intestine between the jejunum and the colon.

Immunosuppressants: Drugs that are given to suppress one or more parts of the immune system. They are used to treat many diseases caused by inflammation as well as to prevent transplanted organ rejection.

Insulin: A hormone that helps to regulate blood sugar by lowering it. Insufficient insulin or lack of sensitivity to insulin can produce the disease diabetes.

Jejunum: The part of the small intestine between the duodenum and the ileum.

Ketosis: An increase of ketones (also called ketone bodies) in the blood. Ketones are chemicals produced by the body from the normal metabolism of fat. For long periods, however, high ketone levels can cause certain problems, particularly in the kidney and liver.

Laparoscope: A tube passed through the skin into the abdomen allowing the doctor to view internal organs (with an attached camera) and perform surgical procedures without the need for a large incision.

Leptin: A hormone produced by fat cells that seems to play a role in the appetite center of the brain.

Lipids: Fats found in the body and measured in the blood. They include HDL ("good") and LDL ("bad") cholesterol as well as triglycerides. Lipids are one of the three main sources of energy for the body and a building block for many cells. The chemical definition is a solid, greasy carbon-based material.

Lipase: An enzyme made by the pancreas that aids in the digestion of fats. Blocking this enzyme with a lipase inhibitor can cause fat malabsorption and weight loss.

Liposuction: A cosmetic surgical procedure to remove fatty tissue under the skin.

Low-density lipoprotein (LDL) cholesterol: "Bad cholesterol." Lipoproteins help to carry the cholesterol from the liver to the rest of the body.

Metabolic syndrome: A medical condition that is a collection of risk factors for serious disease (including diabetes, heart disease, and stroke). The risk factors include high blood (serum) fat/lipid levels, insulin resistance, high blood pressure (hypertension), and elevated markers of infection seen by doing certain blood tests.

Metabolism: The process in which products brought to a living cell are converted into energy and other products that are either used by the cell or excreted.

Mitochondria: The organs within cells that contain genetic material and produce the cells' energy. Mitochondria have been called the "powerhouse" of the cell.

Morbid obesity: At the upper end of the obese weight range. A body mass index of greater than 35 or 40 (this is not fully standardized). Also, massive or extreme obesity

Mutations: Permanent changes in genes. May or may not produce changes in the individual.

Noradrenergic drugs: Drugs used in weight control that act on the brain and are stimulating. They are, in the United States, controlled drugs because they can be addicting. They can produce severe side effects.

Obesity: The condition of being heavier (or having a higher BMI) than overweight and significantly heavier than normal weight. Obesity is defined as a BMI of 30 or higher.

Orthorexia: A disease in which a person wishes to eat only healthy and pure foods to the point of malnutrition and even starvation. They may avoid the "wrong" or "unhealthy" foods such as those made from animals or fats or those that have preservatives.

Over the counter: A term used to describe drugs legally sold in the United States without a doctor's prescription.

Overweight: A body mass index of 25 to 25.9, which is greater than the normal weight (or body mass index) but less than the obese weight range.

Placebo: A "dummy" or inactive pill that is given as a comparative agent in a study of an active drug. Placebos should have no positive effect (efficacy) or negative effect (side effects), but they often do.

Post traumatic stress disorder: A psychiatric condition that follows a major traumatic event. A variety of symptoms can be produced including anxiety, fear, flashbacks of the event (which are often very intense), difficulty sleeping, irritability, anger, and excessive reactions to being surprised or startled.

Prader-Willi syndrome: A rare genetic disorder affecting one or more genes on chromosome 15. It is characterized by a difficult birth, poorly developed sex organs in the baby, failure to thrive, excess sleeping, speech delay, overeating and obesity, spine curvature, poor muscle tone, learning disabilities, and other abnormalities. The overeating may be extremely excessive, leading to morbid obesity.

Prediabetes: An abnormality of glucose metabolism and handling that may be a precursor to or early sign of diabetes.

Protein: One of the three main sources of energy for the body. Proteins are also prime building blocks for many of the cells in the body as well as for hormones, antibodies, enzymes, and other key compounds. One gram of protein contains four calories.

Satiety: The perception of fullness or satisfaction with food that has been eaten. It is a signal that no more food is needed.

Satiety index: A measure of how much a particular food produces satiety (or fullness).

Serotonin: A neurotransmitter found in the brain that seems to play a significant role in the control of appetite and certain moods such as depression and panic.

Serotonin-norepinephrine reuptake inhibitors: Drugs that prevent brain cells from reabsorbing certain neurotransmitters, thus allowing these neurotransmitters to remain in the fluid-filled spaces around the nerves.

These drugs have been used in the treatment of various psychiatric diseases, including depression.

Sleep apnea: A disease seen during sleep in which the patient stops breathing for 10 seconds or more causing the patient to wake up.

Slipped cap femoral epiphysis: A rare but serious problem that occurs in children where the top of the femur slips out of its place in the hip bone. It is seen most commonly in obese adolescent children.

Stem cells: Cells in the body that are capable of transforming into different, specialized cells upon certain stimuli.

Stomal stenosis: A narrowing at the junction of two organs or "tubes." In the context of this book, producing some degree of obstruction to the passage of food.

Trans fats: A specific type of fat—usually solid rather than a liquid or oil—that is made by adding hydrogen to liquid fat. Excess trans fats have been implicated in the development of heart disease and other health problems.

Triglycerides: Lipids or fats composed of three molecules of fatty acid attached to one molecule of glycerol. Elevated levels have been associated with the development of serious medical diseases.

Ventromedial nucleus: The part of the brain found in the hypothalamus associated with satiety. Injury to this area may produce overeating and weight gain.

Yo-yo dieting: Also called weight cycling. The repeated loss and then regain of weight.

Index

Index

Index